Nursing at Burford
A Story of Change

Nursing at Burford
A story of change

Alan Pearson

Professor of Nursing, Deakin University, Geelong, Victoria, Australia;
formerly Head, Burford and Oxford Nursing Development Units.

With an Introductory chapter by Jacqueline Flindell, FRCN, Independent
Nursing Consultant; formerly Chief Nursing Officer, Oxfordshire Health
Authority, and Regional Nursing Officer, Wessex

© Scutari Press 1992

A division of Scutari Projects, the publishing company of the
Royal College of Nursing

First published 1992

British Library Cataloguing in Publication Data

Pearson, Alan
    Nursing at Burford—a story of change.
    I. Title
    610.73

ISBN 1-871364-55-8

Typeset by Action Typesetting Limited, Gloucester
Printed and bound in Great Britain by
Billing & Sons Ltd, Worcester

Contents

Preface

The purpose of the Burford study was to introduce a number of practice changes related to a 'new ideology of nursing', an ideology being promoted by some leaders in nursing in a small community hospital in Burford, Oxfordshire. The study was intended to discover whether the practice changes were 'taken'; whether they were beneficial to nursing staff, patients and the local population, as well as other health care workers; and to explore the change process in the hospital itself.

The methods employed were loosely based on an action research framework and additional and complementary methods were developed as the study progressed. In fact, a triangulation of methods emerged and data were obtained through participant observation, staff surveys, a survey of the local population and the use of measurement tools to establish the quality of care. Data were collected before, during and after changes in nursing practice had been introduced at Burford Hospital, as in a traditional before and after design. When new practices were established, an experimental study of sixty-four patients was carried out to compare patient outcomes between those cared for in other hospitals (the control group) and those cared for at Burford Hospital (the experimental group). This experimental component of the study is not included in this book.

Since Burford Hospital is small and some of the methods employed were highly subjective, no final or definitive conclusions can be drawn. However, the multi-method approach identified trends that supported a number of propositions about the new ideology in nursing and its feasibility in practice. The new norms aimed for became practice norms, and the change process developed appeared to be advantageous to both staff and patients. Consumer perceptions of the nursing process altered as a result of the change effort and patient outcomes were superior to those achieved in other hospitals. Some of the findings have been used to generate axioms for change and identify significant developments in beliefs about nursing among nurses and their patients.

The study concludes with proposals made for practice change and recommendations for the direction of future research.

Alan Pearson

ix

Acknowledgements

Specific thanks are due to my academic supervisors, Ed Randall and John Stone; to the staff of Burford Hospital who journeyed through the study by my side as co-researchers; and the patients who were − and are − the sole justification for any attempt to study the provision of care.

A debt of gratitude is owed to Jacqueline Flindell, the Chief Nursing Officer who initiated the ideas for Burford and appointed me Nurse-in-Charge; to Marnee Heal and Malcolm Ross for the risks they took in giving me the needed freedom to explore innovation, and in releasing and funding me to undertake full-time study; and to the staff of the Computer Centre at Goldsmiths College, especially Hilary and Bev.

Thanks are also due to Mary Parke, who originally typed the thesis, and, at Deakin University, to Monika Loving, Liz Hewitt and Simone Togni for their part in typing this manuscript. Miranda Hughes also deserves thanks for editing my PhD text into this present form.

The lengthy list of others who merit explicit thanks must, for the sake of brevity and practicality, remain in my head. The study embodies the thoughts, work and influence of many others than myself, and acknowledgement is made to all who have listened, reacted, acted and generally supported me throughout the period of study.

Finally, my greatest thanks and appreciation must go, as always, to my full-time supporters, Pauline, Andrew and Stephenie, for helping me to carry through an idea without succumbing to the plague of self-doubt.

1 Introduction: setting the scene
Jacqueline Flindell

'A wise man will make more opportunities than he finds'

Bacon

It gives me great pleasure to write the Introduction to *Nursing at Burford – A Story of Change*. It must surely go down in nursing history as the first attempt to set up a nursing development unit.

We must ask ourselves, why Burford, and why such a small hospital? To understand why Burford, it is appropriate to set the project in context with the Oxfordshire Health Authority at that time. The reorganisation of the National Health Service in 1974 created a Single District Area for Oxfordshire, with a population of 500,000. There were five Hospital Management Committees, with county and city medical and nursing services all to be amalgamated under an Area Health Authority, with chief officers newly appointed. Each of the five Hospital Management Committees supported hospitals which had their own traditions. Apart from the bigger hospitals, like the Radcliffe Infirmary, there were twenty-three health centres and nine cottage hospitals with between nine and twenty-four beds, with Wallingford as a newly-built community hospital of fifty beds. Like all reorganisations the budget control systems were being closely scrutinised and those hospitals that were not cost-effective in financial terms were threatened with closure. Burford had nine beds and came under close monitoring, although no action was taken until 1978 – it was a well-loved small hospital and was part of the community. The matron had been in-post for sixteen years and was due to retire. Burford was a problem – but problems can be opportunities! The community nursing services continued to be separate from the hospital, and access to the wards and co-ordination of the service to the community continued to be separate functions.

At this time the Authority held a public meeting in Burford parish church. There were strong local objections to the closure of the

1

hospital, which had the highest cost per patient of all the hospitals, with an occupancy rate of 75 per cent: the hospital provided a service for the few.

REPRIEVE

It was decided to keep the hospital open but to do everything possible to make it cost-effective. As the chief nurse I knew that nursing must have a vital contribution to make. As in all small hospitals, the patients tended to be long-term rehabilitation, with the emphasis more on nursing care than on medical care. My own view was that true nursing with all its problems took place in all community (cottage) hospitals and much must depend on the skill and attitude of nurses if patients were to be rehabilitated, to be cared for at home or to die with dignity.

EVOLUTION OF THE NURSING DEVELOPMENT UNIT

The Authority had already agreed to the appointment of Dr Sue Pembrey as the clinical practice development nurse. This post was the first in the country, and was unique. She was paid the highest available salary next to the chief nurse and her main task was to be involved in practical nursing, to apply nursing skill based on research findings, to undertake projects and to be the close adviser to the chief nurse on how the standards and practice of nursing were evolving in Oxford. The main teaching hospitals of the District – The Radcliffe Infirmary, John Radcliffe (newly commissioned in 1979), The Churchill, The Nuffield and Banbury – were all hospitals with a high occupancy, and those in the centre of Oxford were concerned with medical treatment with a high-tech approach. The pressure on beds created problems because of the inability to discharge long-term patients whose principal needs were nursing care.

Alan Pearson had just finished his nursing degree and was looking for a job. He came to see me for an informal interview. Why not develop a nursing unit whose sole purpose was to be a centre of excellence in the art and science of nursing? There was no extra money, but the retirement of the matron at Burford Hospital created a vacancy and an opportunity.

Nobody could be more informal than Alan! He had a very 'laid-back' style and I remember thinking, can I take the risk of appointing a male nurse to a Cotswold town like Burford? He was not the traditional image of a matron. We had a most enjoyable hour's discussion on what my vision of the hospital would be, namely a nursing development unit. Getting to know Alan and what his ambitions were was somewhat difficult because of his casual style. He was not keen on management; I explained that it was necessary for him not only to manage a hospital of just nine beds, but also to undertake the public relations role, to work with the League of Friends and to get on with the doctors. This was new ground for Alan. The more I got to know him, the more I saw that he had hidden depths and that, with support from the Divisional Nursing Officer, Marnee Heal, he would be successful. Alan is a naturally creative thinker and seized every opportunity to use the situation to enable Burford to become a nursing practice development unit. During his initial interview we discussed his undertaking a survey of his staff to provide him with a knowledge-base on what they thought about nursing at Burford. How valuable that survey was to be for his research!

One thing a manager has to do is take risks in order to try to achieve a vision. It is not easy for a newly-appointed nursing officer to plough a new field, so the support of colleagues and management is of the utmost importance. I was very conscious of lack of financial support for what was an evolutionary, exciting concept but, nothing daunted, Alan set to. He converted the flat above the hospital into a small unit and invited the community nurses to join the team; so gradually the nurses became a more effective service to the community, working as a team and communicating information to each other and to the community.

ACTION RESEARCH

This research may be described as small, it is true, but its quality and design has produced a piece of work which other nurses can repeat and build upon. Indeed, this has already happened, as we see the mushrooming of clinical nursing development units. The research also justifies the investment in higher education for nurses, where the application and combination of imagination and disciplined thinking can benefit patient care. In my view, nurse managers have a duty to help and encourage such innovations.

Some nurses have stated that there is little to see at Burford when they have made a visit for a study day. The success of Burford is the 'octopedal' way in which nurses become their own ambassadors and inform others through the nursing press. It is the attitude and quality of care being generated, which cannot be measured in one visit.

This piece of research sets out a planned method of implementing change and then evaluating what happened. The success of this change should be measured over five and ten years. If nurses believe in the change, it will survive. I am very confident that nurses, given the opportunity, will wish to sustain a more systematic approach to care. Not only will the nursing profession begin to mature by the practical application of nursing research, but patients will be the recipients of 'quality nursing care' which the profession will be able to justify in any forum.

CHANGE AGENT

Alan correctly reviews the literature concerning many existing attitudes (pp.13 – 16); the task-oriented approach is well documented and it is research such as this that will help to change attitudes. Alan was not only the researcher in this project but also the nursing leader and manager; in reviewing the literature he discovers himself in a unique position and says to himself – will it work? By studying action research methods (Lewin, 1946; Clark and Hockey, 1979) he eventually chose the method advocated by Denzin (1970) (p.30) and so involved all the staff. He clearly sets out his method of approach (p.32) and was conscious of interpreting the information through his own understanding and has studied the work of Konig (1973), Flintstead (1970) and Scott (1979). Inevitably, however vigorous his intentions are, there must be some subjective recording; this type of research is not scientific. I am confident that, in knowing the background and the individual researcher, readers will be convinced by its presentation method and outcomes. The unit and its operational policies are now being reproduced in other parts of the country prior to the publication of this research.

MEASURING QUALITY

The choice of Qualpacs demonstrated that Alan felt that nurses should measure the quality of nursing care. This becomes of greater significance when non-nurses begin to look at the 'skills mix' of staff giving direct patient care. Only nurses can really observe and measure multifunctioning nursing activities; masking, multi-tasking and substitution described by Jennifer Hunt ('Activity balance', *Nursing Standard*, 11 July 1990). Nursing standards also become measurable by peer-group review, and it is this bottom-up approach which will ultimately demonstrate quantifiable nursing activity and the skills necessary to undertake appropriate tasks. It is not my role to comment on every detail of ،the research, but undoubtedly the hierarchy of nursing management has an important role to play. The chief nursing officer may have a vision of where nursing should go, but to get to that vision nursing has to change, and implementation must take place by those at the operational level. This can be helped by a patterned nursing structure which allows for close communication and understanding, and encourages changes to occur. This did not happen immediately in Oxford, but it did become nursing policy in 1981 and was approved by the Authority in 1982. The policy now continues within the John Radcliffe Hospital and in other parts of the District. The senior sister/charge nurse is directly accountable to the most senior nurse manager of the unit. I look forward to the day when the senior sister/charge nurse is as valued in salary terms as the most senior managerial nurse. Both are of the utmost importance in providing satisfactory quality of care and leadership. The senior sister/charge nurse in a 'flattered structure' is concerned not just with managing a ward, but must in addition have a personal assistant to undertake non-nursing administrative tasks. The senior sister is then able to spend more time with 'hands on' patients and teaching. This new role of the senior sister again changes when primary and associate nursing is introduced (*Nursing Times*, 12 November 1986, p.29). The Institute of Nursing at the Radcliffe Infirmary, directed by Dr Sue Pembrey, is already undertaking research in this area (*Nursing Standard*, 1 August 1990, p.52). I believe there will be interesting and appropriate findings of the role of the new senior sister.

The nursing development unit in Burford has become a resource centre for nursing in Oxford and has very close links with the Institute of Nursing. It is only by close clinical links that such units thrive; Oxford leads the way.

The Department of Health will find this piece of research important in political terms because it demonstrates that nurses are capable of affecting the outcomes of patient care when given the opportunity, supported by management, and appointing the right senior nurse to lead, i.e. directing staff to want to change and measuring the outcomes.

'The research demonstrates that consumer perceptions of the nursing process altered as a result of the change effort, and patient outcomes were superior to those achieved in other hospitals.'

Jacqueline Flindell FRCN

2 Burford Community Hospital

The initial idea for carrying out a process of change at the Burford nursing development unit arose out of a number of events which, together, suggested that it should be done.

First, after observing direct patient care in a previous study, I developed the desire to change some of nursing's less positive attributes in reality, rather than through exhortation. Second, as a result of talking and working with 'ordinary' clinical nurses, I realised that the current major drive to encourage nurses to adopt a number of popular changes emanated from academic nurses who were not clinically involved in patient care. Third, the opportunity to do something practical arose when I was offered the post of nursing leader in a small community hospital unit at Burford, which was regarded as 'behind the times', a 'problem', and which needed either to change or to be forgotten. And finally, having worked through these ideas, I discovered that little knowledge or practical information was available to help in the change process I wanted to embark upon.

These four factors led to my attempts both to bring about change in the small hospital concerned and to explore systematically, and eventually report on, what changed, how the change occurred and what the effects were. The study began as an attempt to address four basic questions:

1. Could the changes currently being advocated by nursing's academic elite be implemented in an 'ordinary' unit?
2. If they could be implemented, how would the role of the change agent (in this case myself) develop?
3. What effect would such practice change have on the nurses' perceptions of their roles; consumer perception of the nurse's role; other occupations in the health team; and on patients subjected to the new norms?

4.　If the new norms were possible and had positive effects, what
　　implications would this have for health service provision?

The hospital at Burford offered an opportunity to examine how its
staff would approach the introduction of new norms; the effects of
these new norms; and the process of change as it occurred. Although
the study could only produce findings valid for this specific unit, the
issues with which it was concerned were universal, and lessons can be
learnt from such exercises even though the specifics of the setting
differ. Hospitals, and departments within them, vary widely, but the
ideologies of health workers in western society are similar. Changing
the norms in any nursing team is likely to be a process that shares
many similarities irrespective of the specific unit.
　　A review of the literature suggests that there is some dissatisfaction
with nursing, both from the point of view of those who are the
receivers of its services, and from nurses themselves in terms of their
role in the health care system. A major drive to promote radical
changes is apparent, but little is reported on how this can be brought
about, or on whether or not it ultimately has advantages to patients or
nurses.
　　The purpose of the project at Burford Hospital was to generate and
implement advocated changes and to use a combination of research
methodologies initially to answer the following questions:

1.　Could the changes in nursing currently being advoated be
　　implemented in an 'ordinary nursing unit'?
2.　What effect would the implementation of such changes have on
　　nurses' and consumers' perceptions of nursing?
3.　What effect would the changes have on patient care?

It was also hoped that the study would be able to describe the process
of change and the role of the change agent, and that this part of the
study would present hypotheses to be tested as the study progressed.
　　Answers to the above research questions were required in order to
establish whether or not the energy needed to implement change was
worth expending and, if it was, in what directions change could be
pursued. The open-ended, developmental part of the study was seen
to be crucial, because answering only the basic questions would
assume that the social setting of nursing was predictable, whereas I
believed that additional hypotheses would arise from the study area
rapidly and that testing them would be important in answering the
research questions satisfactorily. Should the findings demonstrate
that advocated changes were of value, I would continue the pursuit of
the new ideologies in nursing. The description of the change process
and new concepts generated and tested would serve to give direction

to other health care teams in planning and implementing changes, and may be of use to policy-makers in the provision of health services.

The overall purpose of the study was thus seen to describe a story of change, and to describe the process and effects of introducing new norms into a nursing unit.

BURFORD COMMUNITY HOSPITAL

Burford Community Hospital is situation in Burford, a small rural town in Oxfordshire with a population of 1,500. Burford itself boasts of having had a hospital for 600 years (Oxfordshire Health Authority, 1978; Moody and Moody, 1983). A cottage hospital was founded in 1868, and was moved to its present site, a building erected through public subscription, in 1902. It became part of the National Health Service in 1948, and since that time there has been a number of attempts to close it, on both economic and policy grounds, when the centralisation of services on District General Hospital sites was a political issue in the 1970s.

A working party paper prepared for the hospital's management team in 1978 reported that medical care was provided by the local general practice of two doctors and that the nine beds at the hospital had an average occupancy of 85 per cent in 1977. A full-time resident matron and 8.5 whole-time equivalent nurses provided nursing care. In addition, there were seven ancillary staff. A 24-hour emergency service for minor injuries was provided and there were out-patient clinics in physiotherapy, chiropody and orthopaedics. A total of 147 outpatients was seen in 1977. An average of four patients spent the day in the hospital each weekday, joining in-patients, in an attempt to provide a day-patient service.

The figures for 1980 (the year preceding commencement of this study) are similar to those for 1978, although bed occupancy for 1980 was only 75 per cent. Approximately 4,000 patients were registered with the local medical practice (consisting of three general practitioners in 1980), 730 (17.5 per cent) of whom were over 65 years of age and 300 (7.1 per cent) over 75. Of all admissions in 1980, 87.5 per cent were over 65, and 61.8 per cent were over 75. Most admissions were elderly people who required medical or nursing care to overcome acute problems; holiday relief stays; and patients for terminal care. Patients registered with other local practices (one in a village 5 miles from the town, and another in a village 7 miles away) were occasionally admitted, although this was discouraged.

Katzmann (1977), reporting on a survey of Burford and its surrounding villages in relation to health care provision, noted that the local people were vehemently defensive about 'their' hospital and that they:

> felt fairly unique in being a relatively small town which had its own hospital, built and supported by very considerable generosity from local people (over £30,000 donated in the last six years) and which met local needs admirably. Furthermore, the hospital had a far greater effect than simply providing care for patients in nine beds. It was part of ... [the town] and provided visible finite evidence of compassion and care given with generosity to local people when ill or suffering.

The original cottage hospital had been established by a well-known local doctor, and his descendants had carried on the attachment. One of the doctors, still in post in 1980, was part of this family. The local populace associated with this handing down of a local resource. Moody and Moody (1983), local residents writing about Burford, give detailed information about the hospital and its history but despite frequent references to medical involvement, they at no point refer to nursing staff or ancillary workers.

The matron of sixteen years retired in 1980. After much debate by the health authority officers they decided to recruit a replacement who had the capacity to develop the hospital, in terms of its nursing service, because at that time the hospital was seen to be uneconomical and its general ethos to be outdated. My application was approved, and I began work as the nursing officer in September 1981.

3 | Changing nursing

The basis of the study framework was formed by a literature review I undertook in the early stages of research. As each phase of the study developed and I became more involved in working at Burford Hospital, it became apparent that there were more specific needs, which required ongoing searches and reviews of the appropriate literature. To highlight the developmental nature of this study, I have presented the literature specific to each phase in the relevant chapters rather than all in this chapter, which is more of an overview.

DEFINING HEALTH

Being 'healthy' is a right of every individual says Mechanic (1975), but achieving such a state in modern society is becoming less and less possible for every member.

'Health' as a term is in itself ambiguous, for it varies in meaning from one society to another, and from one individual to another. Dunn (1961) describes health as 'a state of being, a passive adaptability to the environment', and Engel (1962) asserts that health exists when:

> [T]he organism is sucessfully adjusting in its environment and is able to maintain this state free of undue excitation, capable of growth, development and activity in an integrated and effective sense. . . . This is an active dynamic process taking place in the face of an ever-changing environment. There is continued need for adjustment and adaptation to maintain this state in the face of tasks imposed from the outside or from within the organism itself.

While both of these definitions present a concept of health related to, but not dependent upon the absence of disease, western society frequently views health in relation to disease (Friedson, 1975). The medical model of health is based on the concept of physiological homeostasis. Homeostasis refers to the maintenance within the body of a constant internal environment for cellular survival. Disease – the opposite of health – is a state of imbalance of one or more of the components on the internal environment. Thus the medical/ biological model sees health solely as the absence of disease.

The validity of such assumptions is frequently questioned by social scientists. Field (1972) asks if health is an objective state defined by physicians, or whether it is more a subjective state as perceived by individuals about themselves and influenced by societal values. He sees illness as a form of deviation from social norms, and that it is defined socially in human interaction surrounded by social acts. Friedson describes this deviance as 'conduct which violates sufficiently valued norms'. Like the literature written from a medical standpoint, much of the sociological literature on health tends to define what is not health in order to point towards what is health. Although Friedson (1975) sees the health care system as primarily a mechanism of social control to ensure isolation and treatment of ill members of society, he argues that it is not inevitable that this should be so. Tiffany (1977) purports that health care itself can focus its activities towards promoting the 'state of optimum capacity' to perform effectively those 'valued tasks' of Parsons' (1951) definition of health.

Helt and Pelikan (1975) assert that, currently, health care systems rarely aspire to providing the service suggested by Tiffany and that they concentrate on advancing the interests of professionals or managers. Mechanic (1975) acknowledges that health care involves the promotion of appropriate environmental considerations such as standards of living, education sanitation, availability of nutrients, etc. He asserts that 'good health' only peripherally depends on curative medical acts provided by doctors. Yet, when such expertise is required, Tiffany (1977) notes that:

> to a person in need of the repair services of the hospital with its array of health occupational groups, the quality of hospital care assumes a sudden importance. This is doubly so in the present less than ideal health care system geared as it is to the economic and political interests of health professionals practising hospital-based curative medicine.

Norris (1979) argues for a change in direction in health care, emphasising its role as an enabler of 'self-care'. Levin *et al.* (1979) define self-care as a 'process whereby a lay person functions on his/her own behalf in health promotion and prevention, and in disease detection and treatment'. Norris suggests that the idea of self-care first appeared among health care consumers in the 1960s, beginning with anti-professional and anti-intellectual sentiments, and a desire to return to a way of life that had an emphasis on 'being human, respecting and giving'. She asks: 'but was this really anti-intellectual, or simply a reaction to materialism and mechanistic practices?' Radical writers support the concept of self-care in all spheres, including health care. Illich (1975) describes how increased professionalism in health care has led to the point where significant levels of human suffering are the very result of the professional practice of medicine – iatrogenesis. He comments:

> Once society is so organised that medicine can transform *people* into *patients* because they are unborn, newborn, menopausal, or some other 'age at risk', the population inevitably loses some of its autonomy to its healers.

Those commenting on the growth of the power of medicine, particularly within the field of mental illness (Szasz and Hollender, 1956; Scheff, 1974), stress how the professional worker has the power effectively to remove the individual's right to autonomous decision-making for highly tenuous reasons, while other social theorists emphasise how professional power can be exerted to make compliance with professional values through societal pressure (Goss, 1963; Goffman, 1963; Field, 1972; Zola, 1975).

Norris (1979) emphasises that self-care fundamentally affirms that people and families must be allowed 'to take the initiative, to take responsibility, and to function effectively in developing their own potential for health'. The role of both the health service and its populace of health care workers is then seen to be one of promotion of self-care, through the provision of adequate human and physical resources so that the consumer can achieve self-care, or can act as self-care agents for those who at present are, or are no longer able to be, independent.

NURSING IN THE HEALTH CARE SYSTEM

Nurses are everywhere! They are present in all areas of the health care system – in hospitals, in the community, and within general practice and they 'are present at the birth and death of most of us and could be considered the worker bees of the system' (Tiffany, 1977). The role of the nurse, however, remains unclear. There are still no widely accepted views on what nursing is, who should nurse, when, where and whom (McFarlane, 1980a). Furthermore, despite nurses constituting the largest occupational group in the health service, they are effectively excluded from decision-making, and are seen as being subservient to the medical fraternity (Friedson, 1975). As long as the system revolves around the medical model of:

$$\text{Diagnosis} \rightarrow \text{Treatment} \rightarrow \text{Cure}$$

nursing will continue to be subservient, and be forced to play a less than satisfactory role in decision-making for client needs. There is a growing amount of evidence that nursing does operate on this model, working in a highly routinised way, resisting patient involvement and encouraging patient conformity to the established rules.

McFarlane (1980a) argues 'that the caring role of the nurse has been so neglected' that it needs in-depth expansion as well as the development of a nursing model of care, which she sees as:

$$\text{Assessment} \longrightarrow \text{Help} \longrightarrow \text{Self-care}$$
(of self-care   (assistance, etc.)

ALL IS NOT WELL IN NURSING

As is typical of all organised occupations, nursing has been exhorted to 'change' by its leaders at least since the emergence of Florence Nightingale in the 1850s. Contemporary leaders still enthusiastically urge nurses to pursue changes that reflect the current ideologies. For the last twenty years, emphasis has been made on the need to move away from the established pattern of practice based on routinisation, allocation of tasks and adherence to management and medical models, to a pattern based on meeting the individual needs of the consumer and focused on professionalisation of the nursing role to allow for autonomous practice.

Davies (1976) suggests that in nursing physical care is ranked predominant to psychosocial care and it has become subject to rule-following, standardisation activity and a clear nursing hierarchy with firm allocation of supervisory responsibility. The literature suggests that nurses appear to welcome routinisation. In Britain, the General Nursing Council for England and Wales (nursing's governing body until recently) declared in the 1940s that routine work was of value and a source of satisfaction to the nurse. The recommendations of the Salmon Committee (1966) emphasise standardisation and rule-following, and create a hierarchy to achieve this.

Such standardisation is an effective way of avoiding some of the stress and anxiety inherent in the nurses' work and helps to maintain 24-hour cover when facing high staff turnover and assimilating part-time staff. The pervasive routinisation in clinical care is partly, suggests Menzies (1960), a social defence set up by the hospital nursing services 'to protect its members against the stress arising from their work'. Rigid routines are imposed to remove the need for stressful decision-making and nursing schools socialise students into valuing routine and in performing their role in an impersonal manner without problem-solving or creative thought. Most nursing schools suggests Stein (1978), are highly disciplined, inculcate subservience and inhibit deviance. A fear of independent action results and the clinging to hierarchical support systems becomes a needed and appreciated activity.

Davies (1977) points out how the heavy reliance on nurses as teachers and the protection of student nurses from external influences act as a strong and effective socialisation influence to preserve the rule of routinisation. It transforms current work practices into valued work practices and removes a great deal of uncertainty from the work.

Studies of services for long-stay, chronically ill patients elaborate on routinisation and rule-following. Such services rely heavily on the orderly and auxiliary grades of nurses who are more likely to have a custodial approach to care (Stannard 1973; Williams, 1974). Williams suggests, however, that in spite of access of knowledge of more enlightened approaches, the preoccupation of trained nurses with the more technical and clinical aspects of nursing care may render them as far from treating patients as fellow human beings as the most strictly custodial orderly.

The self-suppressing syndrome of institutionalisation characterised by apathy, resignation, dependence and depersonalisation is now generally recognised, following the work of Goffman (1968). The evidence is that many nurses adopt impersonal attitudes towards patients. Cohen (1964) argues that 'in general, hospital patients have no rights, no dignity, no status'. Chapman (1979) comments that the sick person is expected to yield or to conform, to acknowledge hospital rules and policies even though originally formulated for individuals whose status may have been very different from theirs, and the patient usually conforms because of the perceptions that sanctions may be applied.

Nurses seem obsessed with meeting physical needs and ignoring other needs. Intimate physical handling preoccupies staff to too great an extent and predisposes them quite spontaneously to exaggerate the general dependence of patients. Speed and efficiency are often more important factors than independence; thus patients are unintentionally socialised into dependency. Support through listening and empathising has been found to be sadly lacking in nursing care (Wood, 1979; Faulkner 1981) and the promotion of independence through teaching is apparently almost non-existent.

Patients themselves concur with the view that nurses are obsessed with the performance of tasks associated with physical care and the support of medical regimes, and that they do not fulfil expectation as the humanisers of the health care system. Many studies have reported large numbers of patients who mention communication problems, in one case, it was 86 per cent of respondents (Raphael 1969). Reynolds (1978) found dissatisfaction about information received in general surgical wards and Eardley *et al.* (1975) found education for patients with a chronic disability to be regarded as totally inadequate. Stockwell (1972) reports that patients involved in her study would have liked more opportunities to talk with nurses, but knew that they were 'too busy'. Nursing is heavily criticised in the Royal Commission on the National Health Service (1979) with 88 per cent of those studied regarding paramedical workers as being 'considerate' to them as individuals; 84 per cent with ancillary worker; but only 80 per cent with nurses.

Duberley (1977) argues strongly that carrying out medical orders and carrying out the routine are highly valued and that British nursing generally offers a service based largely on the medical diagnosis; the 'consultant's and/or ward sister's preference'; and the ward routine which are strategically placed in each ward. Ward sisters do attempt to plan care but the plan is based chiefly on doctors' notes, what the patient says in conversation and the added hospital routines, such as 'B.D. − TPRs, early morning tea and no washing of legs on Sundays (because of staff shortages)'.

The subservience of clinical nurses to doctors and nurses in management positions is well documented in the literature. Since the beginning of this century, nursing has been firmly linked with medicine and largely based in institutions. The historical growth of nursing has led to an adoption of the belief that the role of the nurse is to help the doctor. The massive expansion of hospital care systems beginning in the 1920s furthered this view of nursing and the growth in medical technology demanded the development of a group of workers subservient to the doctors, who would apply and monitor this technology and be the doctors' 'eyes and ears'. The focus of nursing became the same as medicine − to cure − and nurses strove to keep patients in a disadvantaged infantile position and thus dependent.

In areas where cure was not probable, such as in long care units the problematic results of nursing adhering to the medical model became apparent because of the position of care at the bottom of a vertical continuum while cure was at the top. Miller and Gwynne (1972) postulate a 'warehouse' model, which is, in effect, a hospital model imposed on those whose needs cannot be appropriately met by applying the medical model. It involves 'people processing' where cure is reinterpreted to mean the 'postponement of death as long as possible'.

The routine work, subordinate to the work of the doctors, needed to be organised and supervised. As the major setting for nursing practice became a bureaucratically structured organisation and was linked with nursing's military and religious roots, obedience, discipline and loyalty became the emphasised characteristics of the work. The general trends in organisation theory advanced by the proponents of the classical management school filtered into nursing, which adopted facets of 'scientific management' and saw the organisation as a machine demanding that 'things' should be run in an orderly fashion (Perrow 1972). Although this approach began to lose favour in the light of the emergence of the human relations management school in the 1930s, and later, the behaviourally inclined political science view, the highly structured organisation advanced by the 'scientific school' has remained a part of nursing.

The literature thus supports the view that all is not well in nursing (and the health care system as a whole). It is this evidence that nurse leaders use to persuade nurses that they need to change and to argue for specific changes.

WHAT NEEDS CHANGING?

McFarlane (1980b) asserts that the cure-oriented/medical-oriented model, pervasive routinisation and a rigid supervisory structure are inappropriate to nursing in any setting, and that the needs of individuals are not being met. Many nurses support this and give voice to the view that nurses should move from a medical model of practice to a model conceived for nursing through the analysis of what people need when they are ill, dependent or unable to perceive how to achieve health. The recognition by many of the need to reform society's beliefs on the role of women led social theorists to question the subservience of nurses (mainly women) to doctors (mainly men) and to criticise the power of medicine (Szasz, 1961; Friedson, 1975; Zola, 1975). Nurses began to assert themselves and seek equality within the health care team. A number of factors has led to this demand for equality. These include: the changing status of women in society as a whole; the higher status of nurses as reflected by salaries; the enhanced quality of the entry to nurse training; the women's liberation movement; the 'too cosy paternalism' of 'some' doctors; the introduction of a new management structure in nursing (Salmon Committee, 1966); improvement in the quality of nurse training; the increased number of men in senior positions; and the rise in trade union involvement by nurses.

Much of this drive for change in nursing largely emanates from nurses in leadership positions at a national level and those who became academics when nursing departments became established in institutes of higher learning during the 1960s (White, 1982). The national nursing bodies exhort nurses to bring about fairly radical changes in their practice based on:

- reorganising work patterns so that care is given by trained nurses and where accountability to the patient is explicit;
- restructuring of the nursing team so that the hierarchy is 'flattened';
- the development of a close relationship between nurse and patient, and the involvement of the patient in planning care;
- basing practice on a model for nursing which incorporates the concept of holism and clarifies the contribution of nursing to health care;
- the use of a problem-solving approach.

The amalgamation of these concepts is said to constitute a major reform in nursing (Pearson and Vaughan, 1984a) and is frequently referred to as 'The Nursing Process' by a vast array of nursing theorists, and written about frequently in all of the major nursing journals. It can be said to represent the current ideology of nursing held by nursing's elite and leadership, and bringing it about in practice has become the concern of a number of initiatives by policy-making bodies.

However, much criticism has been raised both by nurses writing for the popular nursing press and by individual doctors in the medical establishment. Mitchell (1984), in particular, savagely attacks the growing acceptance of the 'new' ideology, claiming that the concepts are 'jargonistic', 'American imports', and that nurses are attempting to 'progressively exclude doctors from nursing affairs'. Rowden (1984) answers Mitchell's criticisms by offering a patient's perspective. He concedes that nurses must involve other members of the health care team but suggests that perhaps doctors could consult nurses when they anticipate practice change.

Duberley (1977) reports that nurses are strongly resistant to the suggested changes for the proposed ideas challenge 'the type of care that nurses generally provide for their patients', and years of past practice is judged as valueless and bad. Mitchell (1984) asserts that the new ideology should not be promoted until there is evidence to support its usefulness and suggests that the patient's opinions should be the ones sought. Such evidence is in small supply. Meyer (1981) reports some improvement in care of the elderly when problem-solving and allocation of patients to nurses is introduced and Metcalfe (1982), using care indices, reports significantly higher patient satisfaction in a maternity area where the 'new' ideas were incorporated into practice. Although advice on how to introduce change appears in the literature, accounts of it actually being done in practice do not. By 1985, there was still no published evidence to suggest that the new ideology will have a favourable effect on patient outcomes or on the satisfaction of nurses. However, it is also true that no publications exist to demonstrate an unfavourable effect.

THE NEW IDEOLOGY IN NURSING: PRACTICAL MODELS

To change the focus of nursing towards the individual needs of the patient through a model based on an alternative to the medical one, and to change it to a model which alters the nurse/patient relationship, is to challenge the traditional ideology of nursing.

The basic curriculum for state registered nurses in any country is still largely based on a medical model that focuses on body systems and disease modes, with nurses receiving a 'watered-down' medical training. There is much evidence to suggest that nurses value carrying out routine tasks and in some sense, nurses are seen as sub-standard doctors. The Royal College of Nursing (1980, 1981) and Orem (1980) argue that the patient will be better served if doctors alone were to pursue a medical model approach, with its concentration on physiological homeostasis and the diagnosis and treatment of disease and illness. This would enable nurses to concentrate on patients as people and help them to make sense of what is happening by giving support and guidance. Alfano (1971) describes how nurses working to the medical model interpret the doctor to the patient, aided and abetted by the patients themselves who wish for the nurse to translate their problems to the doctor. She argues that the new ideology demands a reorientation towards a different view of the world of the patient – a model developed for nursing.

Roper *et al.* (1983) and Punton (1983) describe how the practical application of a nursing model leads to greater patient involvement and to a broader, 'different' approach to the care of people. These models view the recipient of nursing from a holistic perspective; see the goal of nursing as independence, or 'self-care' (Bennett, 1980) for the patient; and define the educational base needed for nursing as a broad understanding of the physiology, psychology and sociology of human living.

Such a concept in nursing is not, however, reflected in the reality of practice or in the training curriculum for registered general nurses. The ideas inherent in such models may, therefore, be threatening to nurses who have been socialised in highly valuing the ideologies previously taught during training (Pearson and Vaughan, 1984b). Alternatives to the dominant medical model are also fiercely criticised by doctors (Orem, 1980), because the models suggest that the discipline of medicine is not necessarily the only, or even the most important, contributor to health care and therefore that the supremacy of doctors must be questioned.

THE NURSE – PATIENT RELATIONSHIP

The changes promoted by nursing leaders include the advocation of closeness between nurse and patient and the idea of partnership (Pearson, 1983; Punton, 1983). Such change topples the current norms of practice which sees the nurse as one who 'plies a trade' for it emphasises that patients have their own unique abilities and desires, and sees the role of the nurse as one of complementing the patient's uniqueness (Capra, 1983).

At present, nurses often maintain a distinct, impersonal position, and, like other health workers, surround themselves with an 'aura of mystery' (Friedson, 1970). They make use of the depersonalisation opportunities offered by the occupational structure and further enhance this distancing between nurse and patient by developing props and aids, such as the widespread, but unnecessary use of face masks (Roth, 1957). In contrast the 'new' practice orientation demands from its nurse–patient relationship a nurse who is self-aware, able to cope with self-disclosure and who possesses highly developed interpersonal relationship skills.

A comparison between the current norms of nursing practice and these 'new' norms indicates the overwhelming discrepancy between the two. Such a discrepancy suggests that, if the new ideas are to be realised, a major, radical effort of change will be necessary. Furthermore, the question of whether or not these changes actually help the patients and nurses remains largely unanswered.

CHANGING NURSING NORMS

What nurses are allowed and expected to do is intimately defined by the society in which they practise. A changing in nursing then, cannot be contemplated without an awareness of the broader issues of social change itself. In other words, changes in nursing cannot occur in isolation from society.

Early sociological theories of social change were part of global theories of society, sometimes called 'grand' or 'evolutionary' theories. In these models, societies inevitably pass through similar stages through the influence of independent forces. For Durkheim, societies changed from mechanical to organic solidarity as a result of technological advance. For Marx societies passed through several types of class struggle under the influence of economic forces. Such evolutionary approaches suggest that social change is both inevitable and unidirectional, and forms the basis of the left-wing debate over revolutionary and non-revolutionary approaches to communism.

Such theories have been said to be non-humanistic. A sociology that is humanistic 'organises enquiry around the characteristic which defines humanity rather than the physical world, that is "meaning" (Bailey, 1975). Evolutionary theories, in contrast, treat man as 'a passive recipient of his environment (not as a potentially active creator of it)'. Bailey (1975) suggests, however, that neo-Marxist developments of 'alienation' are humanist in that they analyse an aspect of meaning of the world for the individual. The perspective of evolutionary theories, in their view of the whole of society itself, is so broad as to be of little use for the change agent in a particular situation 'while they have an illuminating effect in making sense of history, their light is usually too high up to reveal anything but the clumsiest of objects'.

The structural-functionalist and conflict theories are modern derivatives of the evolutionary theory designed to explain issues in contemporary social change. Since nursing is a practice occupation which is mainly concerned with immediate change, structural-functionalism can be readily applied to such change approaches. If we treat society as analogous to a living organism we can use a systems model which treats 'the phenomena and the concepts for organising the phenomena as if there existed organisation, interaction, interdependency and integration of parts and elements. Systems analysis assumes structure and stability within such an arbitrarily sliced and frozen time period' (Chin, 1966). Bailey and Claus (1975) suggest that a system can be conceptualised 'as a way of getting something done. A system is a way of thinking and acting which analyses and integrates knowledge and information for the purpose of improving performance or producing order. A systems approach involves changing or producing something'.

Systems theory as a tool for analysing social events does have its critics. Bailey (1975) disputes that it can describe social change effectively for this takes place over time but systems models are built upon an 'arbitrarily sliced and frozen time period' (Chin, 1966). Walton (1965) points out how the system approach can be criticised as being philosophically reductionist.

In conflict theories, change is as fundamental to social groups as stability is for systems theories. Conflict for social groups is seen as being the impetus for social change. Stability within the social structure is seen as illusory, representing only the dominance of one social group over another. Change is seen to occur when, due to economic or other forces, the power relationships between different social groups alter. Conflict theorists are the major critics of the systems model of social functioning and they purport to explain the 'actual' social world whereas structural-functionalists only explain the 'observed' rules of social interaction. Bailey (1975) suggests that the analysis of power as the primary social force allows for the greater range of social interaction. For conflict theorists, change depends on power. Where consensus exists power is authority; where there is no consensus, power becomes force.

Table 3.1 Power and interaction

Explanatory power of conflict model	Interation type	Explanatory power of consensus model
Force/power	Revolution Rebellion Stand-off Bargaining Truce	Consensus on ends only
Authority/power	Co-operation	Consensus on means and ends

Source: after Bailey 1975.

Other approaches attempt to describe strategies available to the change agent — the person who institutes planned change. Bennis, Benne and Chin (1966) describe the process of planned change as a 'deliberate and collaborative process involving change agent and client systems. These systems are brought together to solve a problem or, more generally, to plan and attain an improved state of functioning in the client system by utilising and applying valid knowledge'.

Bennis Benne and Chin (1966), therefore, take for granted that 'valid knowledge' exists and that there is agreement, at least between the change agent and the client, over what constitutes an 'improved state of functioning'. The focus of research is the 'deliberative and collaborative process'.

Chin (1966) describes several models that could be used by the change agent; the systems model, the developmental model and the model for changing. Differences between the systems model and the model for changing are in stability, source of change and in the goal of intervention.

Table 3.2   Differences between the systems model and the model for change

	Stability	Source of change	Goal of intervention
Systems model	Structural integration	Structural stress	Adjustment, adaption
Model for changing	Unfreezing parts	Self and change agent	Improvement

While such an approach contrasts the 'passive' system model with the more 'active' model for changing, it is not clear how the model for changing can be used to describe a situation initially, without using, for example, a systems approach.

Benne (1966) using a systems model of social change ('The process of social change is essentially a process of 'dis-equilibration – re-equilibration' within a social system') outlines an approach to problems which will enable an organisation to adapt to its social situation most effectively:

1. Problem-solving should be experimental, involving the sensitisation and institutionalisation of feedback mechanisms.
2. Problem-solving should be collaborative.
3. Problem-solving should be task (and reality) -oriented rather than prestige maintaining.
4. Problem-solving should be educational and/or therapeutic for individual participants involved in the change.
5. Effective and efficient problem-solving requires channels of communication.

Barriers to growth are also identified. These include: suppression of feelings of some parts of the system; narrow time-perspectives; and 'lack of adequate mechanisms for mediation and adjustment of conflicts between parts of the system and between the system and other systems in the environment'.

Thompson (1960) separated conflict within organisations into the three areas of technology, labour force and the work environment. Walton (1965) looks at tactics and strategies of social change when two groups are competing for the allocation of the scarce resources of status, political power and money. He describes a 'power strategy' and an 'attitude change strategy', and goes on to state the dilemmas facing leaders of groups who propose to use both strategies in the social arena:

Table 3.3 Power strategy *vs.* Attitude change strategy

Power strategy		Attitude change strategy
Overstating of objectives	versus	De-emphasising differences
Emphasis on power to coerce	versus	Trust
Threat	versus	Conciliation
Coalition (with third parties against competing groups)	versus	Inclusion (of third parties in common cause with competing groups)

While for consensus theories a major problem is to explain social change for conflict theory the major problem is to explain observed social stability, when divergent theories are thought to exist. Various attempts have been made to bridge the gap between conflict and consensus views. Coser (1958), using an analogy of mechanics, suggests that conflict arises within a society because it is generated by 'friction' within the social system. Dahrendorf (1958) suggests that the analyst of change could use both models in any situation: each would highlight different aspects, but each would be valid within its own framework.

Mauksch and Miller (1981) argue that while considersation of the theories of social change is essential in developing a specific strategy, the change-setting demands individual assessment, using an amalgam of theoretical approaches, and that towing a purist line of applying one theory is not usually effective. They suggest however, that planned change is preferable to random changes *per se*.

STRATEGIES FOR CHANGE

'A master plan for managing and directing the flow of change' is how Mauksch and Miller (1981) define strategy: 'Strategy deals with how the influence from the change agent to the change target is processed' and they differentiate between strategies and tactics. A tactic is defined as 'an activity planned and designed to carry out a portion of the plan aimed at implementing change'.

Chin and Benne (1976) describe three types of change strategies. The rational−empirical approach assumes that people are likely to view change positively and work towards it if they are given the basic facts and empirical information, and if this evidence 'indicates that they will derive some benefit from the change'. This strategy requires a logical argument for change and meaningful communication of the argument and its supporting evidence to those who are to be involved in the change.

The normative−reductive approach believe that 'people have

values, norm and attitudes that influence, if not direct their behaviour' (Archer *et al.*, 1984). Giving the argument and facts to support it is therefore seen to be not enough to persuade those involved to change and this approach demands that the change effort focuses on 'helping people to re-examine their values in the hope that they will come to view situations differently'.

Applying power, often through political or economic sanctions, is power-coercive change, the third approach described by Chin and Benne (1976). Archer *et al.* (1984) report on the effectiveness of a combination of rational–empirical and normative–educative strategies in producing community change, and argue that power-coercion should only be used when all else fails.

Ottoway (1976) lists steps with a non-mechanistic approach based on beginning in a pilot site for change:

1. Contracting / establishing a contract / relationship between change agents and clients.
2. Establish a diagnosis, involving the people who will be expected to change.
3. Design intervention.
4. Implement the intervention via those who have been involved in the development of the contract.
5. Provide training in those skills that appear as deficient as a result of the change.
6. Reinforce the new norms.
7. Replicate in other sites.

Ottoway (1976) outlines succinctly the consultation process in his strategy as well as a number of principles for change. First, he contends that change should start from the 'bottom up' rather than from the 'top' people in the organisational structure. Secondly he argues that change should begin in a pilot site rather than across the organisation as a whole suggesting that the new norms, style and environment should actually be practised and established before replication elsewhere. He next maintains that training should follow change 'rather than beginning with training in order to create change'. Fourthly 'contracting a key' is the 'chief characteristic' of Ottoway's strategy, and revolves around 'contracting on how, what and when' between those at the 'bottom who are to change and those responsible for effecting the change ... rather than some one or other group deciding for all'. He next argues that the strategy must be 'made to order' as the 'particular variable of each organisation is so unique that it can be successful only if it is developed and implemented to fit the intrinsic needs and circumstances of each organisation and if it is a pre-planned package for installation'.

Finally he suggests that establishing criteria to determine what, when and how should derive from the 'felt needs' of the group and organisation. In Ottoway's strategy, the pilot site is ready to replicate itself when the staff involved reject old norms and values the new. New sites need not be exact copies of the pilot site, but will learn from the experiences of the pilot-change programme.

CHANGE AGENTS

Change agents have been defined as 'those people either inside or outside the organisation who are providing technical, specialised or consulting assistance in the management of a change effort' (Beckhard, 1969). Ottoway (1980) asserts that everyone is a change agent at some time in their lives. Mauksch and Miller (1981) says that a change agent is:

> a person in a system ... whose role is to assist members of the system in making alterations in themselves or in the system. The change agent may be a professional from outside the system or someone within the system who acts in some official capacity as a change agent.

Ottoway (1980) develops a taxonomic hierarchy for defining a number of change agents. The change generator converts issues into felt needs for change. Some generators lead the conversion and others demonstrate how they value the conversion of the issue to a felt need. Change implementors implement change after the felt need has been recognised. Change adopters are the mass of change agents. Their task is to adopt the change, and by practising it, make it become the new state of normality. The first to adopt the change are called prototypic adopters. Others then follow on from the prototypic adoption.

Archer *et al.* (1984) associate the change agent with the concept of consultancy, emphasising that acting as a consultant in a collaborative process is the crucial role of change agents whether they are from outside the work group or part of it.

A number of writers argue, however, that the change agent, by definition, must be from an outside agency or employed specifically to effect change. That there is confusion about the role of the change agent is evident and is in need of clarification. Ottoway (1980) argues strongly that the change agent can be a part of the working team, and that managers can effect change and cites the experiences of Gross *et al.* (1971) which support the assertion that change agents are more effective if they become 'catalytic role models'.

AN ECLECTIC APPROACH TO A CHANGE STRATEGY AND AGENCY

Archer *et al.* (1984) argue that change should be 'mutual and dynamic' and focused on collaboration between all concerned. They suggest that such an orientation leads to a situation where all participants experience change:

> because of their experience in the collaborative intersystem, as they receive inputs and feedback from their respective systems, as they are influenced by their environments, and as they live with the consequence of their collaborative efforts.... Change in people and in the systems in which they interact is necessary to bring about whatever change people and their systems desire. Change is not only constant, it is all pervading.

While they emphasise collaboration and consultation, Archer *et al.* (1984) are eclectic in their approach, using any theory or strategical design if it is of use to the change situation. This approach supports the amalgam of varying theories and concepts as a basis for a change strategy for changing nursing.

Reorienting a nursing team in a real practice, setting the focus on the issues which demand changes in nursing and negotiating with the whole social group which makes up a health care team to implement these changes through the use of alternative approaches and social change theories can be reasonably described as an exercise of much complexity!

Aware of the complexity of these assumptions, my work evolved as an attempt to introduce the new ideas to the nursing team, and to study the process and effects of making them the new norms of practice, and to do this as painlessly as possible to all involved (myself included!). It was clear from the very beginning that this would not be easy for I would have to fulfil a number of roles, not all of which would sit easily together: not only was I the change agent and participating fully in the change process but I was also trying to maintain my role as nursing leader, which included a degree of organisational responsibility and decisions of authority.

The future history of nursing must include references to the Burford experiment. It was the first effort to try to correlate the attainments of nursing academia and practical nursing, while not ignoring the experience of nurses trained in the well-tried apprenticeship scheme, but rather building on the knowledge and practical experience hitherto not brought into a disciplined way of thinking in relation to nursing.

4 The Burford study

A TAILOR-MADE RESEARCH DESIGN

It was clear that the needs of the Burford Community Hospital should determine how these complex questions and aims of the last chapter could be researched, rather than making the hospital fit into standard methodologies.

Was 'quantitative, orthodox method, with its ready acceptability and precise findings' (Bond, 1978) possible or even desirable? Would a qualitative approach be more meaningful when the subjects are people with diverse personalities, roles and experiences? Could I do research with these people rather than on them according to the new paradigm advocated by Reason and Rowan (1981)? Since the potential sample field of Burford Community Hospital was small, the traditional one method/one design approach, with its emphasis on producing findings of statistical significance was not seen as being suitable. I planned to base the steps of the study loosely on an action research model, modified by the incorporation of other designs and methods.

Under the old orthodox paradigm, research was believed to be totally objective, but Reason and Rowan suggest that under the new paradigm, research is objectively subjective. They criticise orthodox methodology because of its model of the person, where people are only seen as units of a research design, isolated from their normal social contexts and reduced to a set of variables. Reason and Rowan (1981) argue that the new paradigm, although very much opposed to its antecedents, is a synthesis of naive inquiry (which is totally subjective) and orthodox research.

Qualitative methods are seen to be crucial to the development of new theories by Glaser and Strauss (1967) in their account of 'grounded theory'. Grounded theory suggests that theory should be grounded in data systematically obtained and analysed through a

27

method of constant, comparative analysis. They argue that there should be more emphasis on generating new theories and less on verifying existing ones.

Lewin (1946) first described 'action research', where the researcher acts as change agent and assesses a current situation, feeds information or procedural change into it and alters present practice accordingly. The results of the intervention are then assessed, fed back to the client group and the cycle begins again.

Because of the nature of this study, action research was felt to be the method on which to hinge the project, although it was anticipated that an orthodox quantifiable approach would be pursued when the study developed. Denzin (1970) argues for a 'triangulation' of research methods in sociological research where different methodologies are applied to one study in order to gain maximum data. Hall (1978) also suggests that sociologists can hope to overcome the intrinsic bias that comes from the single-method, single-observer, single-theory studies if they combine multiple data sources and/or methods. Denzin (1970) further suggests that qualitative data can be used quantitatively and argues that qualitative data produces initial propositions worthy of pursuit, but that quantifiable methods should then be applied to test such propositions.

A FOCUS ON ACTION RESEARCH

Clark and Hockey (1979) describe three types of empirical research: descriptive experimental and action: 'In action research, the researcher's focus is a local situation in which he either wishes to solve a local problem or to evaluate the effects of a specific change involving the people who are part of the situation.' An action approach can also include the researcher as change agent, and the design and study of the action during the problem-solving process. An alternative approach can be where the researcher evaluates change by involving the people concerned in the evaluation by interviewing and observing them and by discussing the objectives of their work with them.

Miller and Gwynne (1972) argue that the people who make up the institution – in their study, a facility for the disabled – have to decide whether or not they will endorse the concept of care suggested by the researcher and the task is then to evaluate the change in such a way that lessons could be learnt from it.

In all approaches, the education of the client is important, and action research and action learning can be identical processes. The major challenge of pursuing an action approach is the double commitment of serving the client(s) and of advancing knowledge at the same time (Rapaport, 1970). 'Action research aims to contribute both to the practical concerns of people in an immediate problematic situation and to the goals of social science by joint collaboration within a mutually acceptable ethical framework.'

Learning and training are seen as crucial elements in the action process by Sanford (1970), whose model is constructed on the five steps of: analysis, fact-finding, planning, execution and evaluation. Originally described by Lewin (1946), action research can be undertaken on individuals and groups or in larger systems such as communities and health services. In the latter, it can be seen as 'planned and tested innovation in social policy'.

Towell (1979) says that social research can be used for confronting the problems that arise during change. The participation needed between the change agent/researcher and the client(s) is emphasised in his strategy. Since the aim of action research is to facilitate the growth and development of individuals and groups, the recipients must be made aware of the programme. As Sanford (1970) says, 'there is no point in planning for people who will upset all such plans as soon as they find out that they have not been permitted to take part in the planning'.

Donnison (1970) argues that the overall aim of the action approach is to bring about social reform. If action research does not achieve reform Donnison says that it could avoid destructive failures of change brought about by other means and therefore add to the repository of knowledge about social change.

Susman and Evered (1978) say that process, rather than outcome, is the aim of action research leading to the development of new knowledge about change in organisations. 'Action research is shown to be able to base its scientific legitimacy in philosophical traditions that are different from those which legitimate positivist science.' They claim that both deductive and inductive reasoning have failed to advance knowledge about the real change process and their understanding.

Action research and the qualitative methodology described by Glaser and Strauss (1967) have some similarities and some differences. As the aims at the beginning are open in grounded theory (Glaser and Strauss 1970), so is the formulation of the problems in action research (Sanford, 1970; Ottoway, 1976). In both these approaches, observation and hypothesising are on-going and interrelated and have a guiding role in the research function (Glaser and Strauss 1970; Susman and Evered, 1978). However, qualitative analysis demands that sampling should continue until saturation, while in action research, a hypothesis may be based on one single event and action then taken. The qualitative researcher analyses with the aim of building theory which can be generalised, and remains an observer although he or she may share part of the life of the subjects. In contrast, the action researcher tries to substitute theory from the change he or she is concerned with, and may be unable to generalise, although the theory may well serve other people concerned with change in a similar setting. Action research has to meet both the needs of the client system and those of the research into what happens in the change, and if it should or should not happen in this way.

I decided to use the strategy of multiple triangulation advocated by Denzin (1970). This meant that the research problem of changing nursing norms was able to be explored from many different methodological perspectives. It seems to be a useful strategy to use alongside the Susman and Evered action research cycle. Not only would such an approach produce a richer exposition, but I also hoped that it would also give more reliable results because the small sample size would render the results of one approach non-generalisable if statistical significance could not be demonstrated. Denzin (1970) lists four types of triangulation:

1. Data triangulation.
2. Investigator triangulation.
3. Theory triangulation.
4. Methodological triangulation.

The basic design was derived from triangulating data theory and methodology in the following way:

1. *Data:* Both qualitative and quantitative data were collected from the local population, the staff and the patients.
2. *Investigator:* As the main investigator and researcher, I used both participant and non-participant observer roles as well as occupying change agent/researcher/co-worker roles simul-taneously. When required, external investigators collected data.
3. *Theory:* The study was based on a framework drawing from a range of concepts both inductive and deductive, which were to be explored rather than a theory to be tested.
4. *Methodological:* A number of methodologies were used: participant and non-participant observation; survey question-naires; direct observation; observer participation; document analysis; manipulation of independent variables to produce experimental conditions; and the exercising of qualitative judgement to rate quality.

In addition to this range of approaches, the hospital staff were fully involved in the research process in their answering of the research questions.

The research design can, therefore, be summarised as multi-methodological, based on the steps of the cyclical action research process, as an operational framework, but expanding beyond that process theoretically. A phased design was constructed, with the first four phases being planned at the beginning of the study, and further phases added as the study progressed.

Phase I: Assessing and establishing objectives

This phase was the diagnostic first step of the action research process, and began six months before I started working at Burford Hospital. It ended when problems were defined or identified, some time after I became a participant observer. This phase included:

1. Collection of base-line data to ascertain:
    (a) attitudes and expectations of nursing of the local population;
    (b) attitudes and expectations of nursing of the unit staff;
    (c) the characteristics of the local community as a whole;
    (d) the quality of nursing care in the unit.
2. Collection of data to ascertain the organisation of the nursing work.
3. A planned programme of teaching for the unit staff to develop a basic understanding of the contemporary ideas suggestive of changing nursing.
4. Collection of data to illuminate the current ideologies held about the work in the unit by its staff.

Part 1 of the phase was carried out before I arrived at the hospital to become part of the staff, and parts 2–4 after this had occurred.

Phase 2: Action planning

Action planning commenced when the Burford staff and I agreed to identify the problems that pre-empted the need to change, and was completed when appropriate courses of action were agreed upon.

Phase 3: Action-taking

Action-taking stated when it was possible to introduce change.

Phase 4: Evaluation

Evaluation included:

1. A repeat of the base-line data collected in phase 1 to evaluate effects of the changes on the staff and the consumers, and in the quality of care.

2.   Analysis and feedback of qualitative data collected throughout
     preceding phases.

Phase 5: Testing hypotheses

This was an additional step to the model described by Susman and
Evered (1978), and was, in effect, an application of an experimental
design to test any hypotheses generated by the action research
process. It was actually a re-entry into the cyclical action research
process, using a more quantitative approach to evaluate further
findings from phase 4. This phase is not reported on in this book,
which focuses on the process of change.

It was not possible to allocate times for these phases at the
beginning of the project because these were dependent on the process
itself, and had to be decided collaboratively between the Burford unit
staff and myself. In the end, the fieldwork for the study lasted for
three and a half years, with the phases lasting as in Figure 4.1. The
'specifying learning' step in Susman and Evered's (1978) model was
seen to be the final discussion of the study.

Phase 1:	Assessed and established objectives
	Researcher outside unit (6 months)
	Researcher part of unit staff (9 months)
Phase 2:	Action planned
	(3 months)
Phase 3:	Action taken
	(11 months)
Phase 4:	Evaluating the change process and outcome
	(6 months)
Phase 5:	Testing the major hypotheses generated
	Experimental design to compare patient outcomes between 'ordinary' nursing unit and unit with 'new' nurses (8 months)

Fig. 4.1   Study design

METHODS

A variety of methods of data collection were decided upon:

1.   A continual collection of qualitative data throughout phases 1–5
     through the use of: process recording of unstructured interviews
     of staff on an *ad hoc* basis when indicated by the events; the
     completion of a daily diary by myself divided in observations

inferences and interpretations; tape recordings of group sessions aimed at discussing the role of the nurse.

2. Questionnaires to ascertain attitudes and expectations of the hospital staff, the consumer population, and to measure the quality of nursing care, to be used during phases 1 and 4 of the study.

3. Questionnaires to test the hypothesis developed in phase 4 to be administered in phase 5. This was not developed until the last phase of the study.

QUALITATIVE METHODS

A major aim of the study was to explore objectively the subjective events of the change process. One aspect of using either the action research methodology or that of qualitative methodology is the need to leave many questions open and to generate questions or hypotheses from what happens. The purpose of collecting subjective data throughout the first four phases of the study was to use it as an account of the events involved to be analysed and classified qualitatively and attempt to make sense of what happened.

The unstructured interviews were recorded with the researcher as participant, and the daily diary was completed at the end of each day, although some entries were made during the day if I felt it was important to commit an observation to writing before it was forgotten, and I was able to withdraw and write at that moment. Konig (1973) says that while observation takes place, so does recognition and what is recognised is partly determined by the observer's structuring of what is seen, in order to understand it in the light of his or her own personal structure. He suggests that this problem cannot be solved technically, but that making rules to write observations and inferences *before* interpreting them is a way of dealing with them. Filstead (1970) emphasises that 'understanding' is the core concept in qualitative methodology, and he and Konig argue that the collector of qualitative data must interpret it through his or her understanding; be rigorous about recording and inferring, and involving the subject before interpreting. In this way, the reporting of the data can be trusted. Scott (1979) says that 'the essence is one of trust that [the researcher's] reporting is seen to be fair and honest'. The actual recording of these data was planned to include the application of these principles to the process recordings and diary entries.

Tape recordings of our group sessions were typed up as transcripts and were later subjected to content analysis and categorisation.

THE QUESTIONNAIRES

Oppenheim (1966) defines a questionnaire as a 'scientific' instrument for measurement and collection of data and not just a list of questions or a form to fill in. He adds, however, that the formulation of questions is a matter of art, not science, and that there are few rules which can be said to be constantly applicable. Common sense, says Oppenheim, is of greater importance.

Using a variety of types of questions suggested by the literature, I developed a questionnaire (Appendix I). I decided to administer it to all members of the staff at Burford Hospital to find out how they felt about nursing. The questionnaire consisted of five sections. The qualified nurses were given the full questionnaire, while the ancillary staff given only section V.

The first section consisted of a modification of the 'rank ordering' of parts of nursing according to the respondents' perception of the nursing role, developed by Anderson (1973). I modified the wording of the questions so that they were more relevant to our hospital. The second part contained ten open-ended questions designed to find out the respondents' involvement in nursing matters generally. The third section contained six brief vignettes and a request about reactions if placed in those situations. The purpose of this was to discover how the respondent felt about power structures within the health team, and how assertive she or he felt within it. The fourth section was designed to assess empathy levels, based on a test of Carkhuff (1969). There were three vignettes, and the respondents were asked to indicate their reactions. The last section contained ten 'sentence completion' questions, similar to those used by Faulkner (1981), to ascertain the perception of the nursing role and of Burford Hospital.

The attitudes and expectations of the consumer population were assessed by their completing a questionnaire containing the ten sentence completion questions of section V. In addition, they answered questions about their previous involvement with both Burford Hospital and other health care facilities.

Attempts to develop ways of measuring the quality of nursing care have been a preoccupation of nursing for some years, and a number of tools designed to do this have emerged in North America. British nursing has, until recently, expended less energy on this task than its American colleagues, but there is now work being done on establishing minimum acceptable standards which could be used as criteria for evaluating care (Royal College of Nursing, 1979a, 1980).

Hegyvary and Haussman (1976) list three areas of practice which may be evaluated: structure, process and outcome. Structure refers to the external conditions which enable nursing to take place; process, the behaviour and acts of nurses; and outcome, the actual results. Mayers *et al.* (1977) argue that patients get better, often in spite of nursing, rather than because of it. Evaluating the structure is said to be of use by Clark (1984), but Pearson (1984) sees such an approach as being a tool to point out the deficiencies of management which will aid an increase in quality, but which is an inadequate way in which to judge the quality of nursing care.

Bloch (1975), Doughty and Mash (1977) and Hover and Zimmer (1978) all agree that evaluating the process is the most important perspective on which to judge quality, although incorporating outcome measures is seen to be also of use. I therefore decided to use the Quality of Patient Care Scale (Qualpacs) scheme, developed by Wandelt and Ager (1974), because it had previously been well tested for reliability and validity.

The Quality of Patient Care Scale concentrates on the process of nursing by observing care directly. It consists of 68 items in the form of a chart, and is arranged in the following six sub-sections:

1. *Psychosocial: individual* (15 items) − actions directed towards meeting psychosocial needs of individual patients.
2. *Psychosocial: group* (8 items) − actions directed towards meeting psychosocial needs of patients as members of a group.
3. *Physical:* (15 items) − actions directed towards meeting physical needs of patients.
4. *General:* (15 items) − actions directed towards meeting either psychosocial or physical needs of the patient, or both at the same time.
5. *Communication:* (8 items) − communication on behalf of the patient.
6. *Professional implications:* (7 items) − care given to patients reflects initiative and responsibility indicative of professional expectations.

Each individual item is accompanied by a concise statement of action and a 20-page 'cue-sheet' gives specific examples of such activities to assist the rate. Two raters together are expected to observe care being given to a small group of randomly selected patients and to score the care using the Qualpacs charts. All interactions with each patient are recorded and may include various nurses of different grades. At the end of the recording, a mean score can be calculated and the numerical score (out of a total of 5) can be equated to a descriptive statement:

1 = poorest care
2 = between

3   =   average care
4   =   between
5   =   best care

The Quality of Patient Care Scale is thus a method of process evaluation applied while real care is being delivered, using direct observation.

By stage 5 of the study, we all agreed that a need still existed to establish whether or not the new norms had had any effect on patients themselves and to test for this experimentally through comparing patient outcomes between those nursed at Burford and at other hospitals where the new norms were not apparent. We decided to interview all of the patients in the study on discharge from hospital, and at the control sites of other hospitals. For this purpose, an interview schedule was developed (Appendix III) and all answers were coded for computation. Although this component of the study is not reported on in this book, the measures used were developed through drawing on the first four stages of the study.

The first part of this schedule obtained basic biographical, medical and social data concerning the subject. Part 2 was adapted from study on stroke patients (Garraway *et al.,* 1980). The purpose was to measure the level of independence in the subject on discharge and to determine the level of dependence on others. This 'dependency index' consisted of a list of common living activities corresponding to a five point scale to indicate the level of dependence in each. An accompanying criteria list clarified the use of the scale to the interviewer.

The third part consisted of closed questions related to a three-point scale intended to assess the subject's general satisfaction with life. This section was based on the 'Life satisfaction profile' developed by Neugarten *et al.* (1961), and used by Luker (1982) in her study of the effects of health visiting on patient outcomes. Part 4 was an adaption of the patient service checklist used by Hall *et al.* (1975) in North America and the adaptions made were in vocabulary. It consisted of 46 statements about the nursing received, to which the respondent was asked to indicate if the statements made were true, untrue or not applicable.

The 'nursing audit' schedules developed by Phaneuf (1976) were used to assess the quality of care as indicated by each patient's record. It is a process-oriented approach for appraising nursing care by retrospective examination of patients' records. Trained nurse-auditors use an audit schedule, structured on seven functions of nursing, for each record. These are:

1.   The application and execution of the doctors' legal orders.
2.   The observations of symptoms and reactions.

3. Supervision of the patient.
4. Supervision of those participating in care.
5. Reporting and recording.
6. The application of nursing procedures and techniques.
7. The promotion of health by directing and teaching.

From these seven functions, fifty components are identified to help auditors evaluate the quality of nursing by 'focusing their attention on the patient rather than on the nursing specialities or the nurses who administer care' (Marriner, 1979). The fifty components are stated in terms of actions by nurses in relation to the patient, and in the form of questions to be answered by the auditors as they review the patients' records.

Part 1 of the schedule elicits basic data about the patient and part 2 consists of a structured chart review schedule. The fifty components derived from the seven nursing functions are posed in terms of questions to be answered by the auditor. In answering each question, the auditor may respond with 'uncertain', and in some items, 'does not apply'. After completion of part 2, the reply to each question is scored and the score is then weighted according to the relative importance assigned to the components concerned. Phaneuf (1976) describes how the weighing system was derived from extensive testing of the instrument.

The final audit score is arrived at by multiplying the total score of individual component scores by a value determined by the 'does not apply' responses, and is equated to one of five descriptive statements:

161 – 200 = excellent
121 – 160 = good
81 – 120 = incomplete
41 – 80 = poor
0 – 40 = unsafe

5 The beginning: Burford as it was

PHASE 1: ASSESSING AND ESTABLISHING OBJECTIVES

The first phase of the study had two objectives. First, within the context of the change and action research process, this phase aimed at establishing what nursing in the hospital was and determining what changes needed to be made. Secondly, within the wider context of the study as a whole, part of the phase also aimed at collecting base-line data about the hospital work to be compared with the results of the collection of the same kind of data at a later stage (phase 4) so that a 'before and after' evaluation could occur.

Phase 1 lasted 15 months, and was clearly divided into two parts. In the first six months, because I was engaged in another project at the opposite end of the country, I was only able to make brief monthly visits to Oxfordshire to liaise with senior managers within the Oxford Health District, and to become superficially familiar with Burford Hospital and its staff. During this time, base-line data were collected and analysed before I became a part of the hospital staff, or had the opportunity to influence the staff and the local population. The next nine months were spent collecting qualitative data, carrying out a planned educational programme and formulating a diagnosis.

The base-line data collected concerned the attitudes of the staff and the community, and a measurement of the quality of care. The lists of the questions asked can be found in Appendices I – II at the end of this book.

THE STAFF QUESTIONNAIRE ABOUT NURSING ATTITUDES

Of the five most important activities that nurses thought nursing involved, four related to physical or medical care and one to

38

psychosocial care, that is, explaining procedures to the patient. This particular activity does, however, relate to a procedure and so can also be perceived as being related to an act of physicality, and if this is accepted, all of the top five activities relate to physical, medical or the 'doing' of care. Four of the five activities thought least important by the nurses concerned psychosocial care, with the one exception being 'conducting the consultant's ward round'. It would seem, therefore, that the qualified nurses value the medically-related and physically-oriented parts of nursing and see psychosocial care as being of less importance. Given the comments of the ninth respondent who did not complete this section, but who commented that 'giving information to the patient about his condition' was not the role of the nurse, and that all of the other respondents ranked it not higher than 8th, this activity was clearly seen to be unimportant.

Nursing as a profession

None of the nurses at Burford subscribed to a nursing journal, although all said that they read those supplied to the hospital; none had attended any courses or conferences in the last year; and none were members of a professional association or trade union. Sixty-six per cent said that they intended to stay in the same job for the foreseeable future; while one said she would like to take a course; one said she would like to 'progress when home commitments allow'; and one said she would like to become a district nurse.

One respondent had had a nursing care study published in the nursing press, and a short story published in a fiction magazine (both in student days). Four respondents detailed specific articles or books they had read during the last year related to their own work, while five made no response.

In professionally-related activities outside work, one respondent worked with the Samaritans, and another was an active member of the Women's Institute.

Assertiveness

These questions were designed to elicit the degree to which a nurse would assert herself in a situation, and how reasoned the reaction would be. The following responses to the five vignettes (see Appendix I) were recorded.

1. This vignette concerned an error in payment of salary, with no forthcoming explanation. All respondents said they would pursue the matter further, with three saying that they would wait until the next month's payment to see if it occurred again before doing so; two

saying that they would insist on an answer being given immediately; and four saying that they would find out more themselves before doing anything. All were thus prepared to assert themselves in this situation.

2.   This vignette concerned a request that the respondent see the divisional nursing officer at a time which would conflict with a previously made arrangement to meet a friend. All of the respondents indicated that the appointment with the friend would be cancelled and the one with the senior nurse kept. One respondent indicated, however, that she felt angry that she would do this, while four said that the appointment with the friend would be easier to put off. The group was apparently less willing to assert themselves in relation to the nursing hierarchy than in the issue of their own pay.

3.   The doctor discharging a patient home when the nurse felt it was wrong to do so was the subject of this vignette. One respondent indicated strongly that the issue was one where nurses should be involved, while the other eight all said that they would follow the doctor's orders. Of these eight, however, three said that they would take other steps to involve the family and/or support services. Five also said that they would make some overture to the doctor to change his mind – one, for example, saying, 'Making a further appeal to the doctor on social grounds', but all added that they would fall in with the doctor's eventual decision, for example, 'if this fails to move [the doctor], go ahead with the discharge'. Like the senior nurse involved in the second vignette, the doctor too appears to be someone who was unlikely to be challenged by this group of nurses.

4.   The next vignette involved being pushed out of a bus queue and asks for a response to the situation where the respondent fails to get on the bus as a result. Six said that they would explain what happened to the bus conductor in the hope that he would expel the person who pushed in; one said that she would get on the bus and refuse to get off and two said that they would wait for the next bus 'to avoid a scene'. The majority therefore appear to be prepared to assert themselves logically in this wronged situation.

5.   The final vignette in this section concerned another nursing colleague at work who asked the respondent to admit a patient while she 'did the pharmacy', even though the respondent was off-duty. All said they would not admit the patient and that they would tell the other nurse that the admission was more important than the pharmacy order.

The results broadly suggest that this group was reasonably assertive, but that they were unlikely to assert themselves to those who they considered to be superior to them, and that both the divisional nursing officer and the doctor fell into this category.

Section IV

This section assessed empathy levels. Based on Carkhuff's (1969) empathy rating scales, his criteria were used to assess how much the nurses' attempts to identify with the subjects in the vignette (see Appendix I). Eight of the nurses made responses which showed no attempt to empathise and which concentrated on the organisational aspects of the story. For example, explaining to the domestic who had problems at home and who made a telephone call during work-time, that 'telephone calls were not allowed, and that this should be done after work'. In the cases of the patient in casualty with bruises inflicted by her husband, and of the patient in the ward who was disruptive, a reading of the rules was suggested and referral to the doctor seen as the solution to both. Only one nurse attempted to understand the feelings of the subject of the vignette.

Section V

The answers to these ten sentence completion questions (see Appendix I) were categorised by an external judge. The results suggested that the qualified nurses saw their role as one that supported that of the doctor, with 78 per cent (n = 7) saying that nurses carried out the medical orders, and the characteristics of a 'good nurse' included such personality traits as 'caring' and 'cheerful' and the ability to meet patients' needs. The notion of the 'poor' nurse was related to attitudes such as caring, interest or 'thinking about the patient', rather than to competence or intelligence; and a 'good, basic education' was regarded as the educational requirement for nursing. This group liked Burford Hospital's atmosphere of friendliness and its closeness to the community but disliked, in particular, the then prevailing practice of looking after the day patients within the ward areas.

QUESTIONNAIRE: UNTRAINED NURSES

All of the untrained ancillary workers returned the questionnaires, which consisted of the sentence completion questions of section V of the qualified nurses' questionnaire. The results were similar to those of qualified nurses.

QUESTIONNAIRE: CONSUMERS

One hundred and sixty-two questionnaires were returned, giving a response rate of 81 per cent. Many of them were accompanied by either a separate letter or a lengthy comment on the questionnaire itself. Twenty-seven (16.2 per cent) strongly defended Burford Hospital and its nurses, and stated how they abhorred the 'talk of closing the hospital down'. Five respondents also criticised the questionnaire itself, one suggesting that the National Health Service should spend its money on patients rather than on 'silly surveys' and one suggesting, having noted that I was both a man and a nurse, that 'this is what happens when men start being nurses'!

The consumers were predominantly female and 25.6 per cent were over 65. From the stated occupation on the questionnaire (or, if the women stated 'housewife', her spouse's occupation) the social class was determined according to the classifications of the Registrar General. The majority of consumers were in social class 3, of skilled workers, although all classifications were well represented.

Only 24 respondents (15 per cent) had ever used the hospital, and three (2 per cent) were regularly attending the hospital. Sixty respondents (37 per cent) said that they had attended other hospitals for treatment which they felt could have been given at Burford Hospital.

X-ray	11
Accident treatment	19
Maternity	3
Surgical operation	1
Heart attack	1

Fig. 5.1 Treatment received at other hospitals which respondents felt could be given at Burford.

The overall picture of nursing from the results appeared to be that the 'good' nurse has the 'right personality' (caring, cheerful, unselfish) and that this is more important than intelligence or education. Although respondents saw a difficulty in self-care as the factor that determines a need for nursing, the work of nurse was seen to be the carrying out of doctors' orders, but respondents thought nursing was best taught by other nurses. A 'poor' nurse was seen as one who is uncaring and who did not have a vocation.

Rather than the quality of care, the best things about Burford Hospital were perceived to be convenience, handiness, homeliness and friendliness. The worst was its small size. Many comments about the constant threat of closure were made here, and nine respondents complained that it was associated too much with the local two-man medical practice and that it should cater for the people of the district, not the people registered with a specific general practitioner. Nursing in the hospital was seen to be different from other hospitals in that it was possible for it to be personal, rather than catering for an ever-changing patient population in a large, acute hospital. The results suggested that the population was fiercely defensive about Burford Hospital, seeing it as small and friendly, but lacking facilities, and its role as predominantly medical.

QUALITY OF CARE ASSESSMENT

Four day staff and two night staff were observed nursing three female and two male patients over a period of five hours.

The overall Qualpacs score was calculated to be 2.6 out of a maximum of 5, with the care for the female patients scoring 2.5, and for the males, 2.8. Psychosocial care related to the individual was assessed to score 2.8 overall, while group psychosocial care was scored at 2.2. The nurses' (all of whom were female) response to the female patients within the group setting scored only 1.3, compared with 2.7 for the males. The results showed that physical care scored the highest, with 2.9 out of 5. General care scored 2.5, communications, 2.7, and professional implications, 2.0. Since none of the sections achieved the score of 3, which is regarded as 'average care', the overall mean score suggests that care was below average.

Table 5.1 Mean Qualpacs scores

	Male patients	Female patients	All patients
Psychosocial: individual	2.9	2.7	2.8
Psychosocial: group	2.7	1.3	2.2
Physical	2.9	2.9	2.9
General	2.7	2.3	2.5
Communications	2.7	2.7	2.7
Professional implications	2.5	1.8	2.0
Mean total	2.9	2.7	2.8

As far as the scores for individual members of staff were concerned, both of the nursing auxiliaries had an overall mean score which reflected above-average care, while two of the four qualified nurses scored below 3.

Table 5.2 Individual nurse's scores

Nurse	Mean score
Night staff nurse	2.6
Night auxiliary	3.1
Sister	3.0
Staff nurse	3.4
Enrolled nurse	2.6
Auxiliary nurse	3.3

Anecdotal notes made by the observers pointed out both the positive and negative aspects of observed care. While some individual nurses clearly tried to give both individual and group psychosocial care, some did not, and few examples of regarding the patients in the hospital as a social group were observed. Few examples of communication on behalf of the patient, actions which reflected initiative or responsibility, or evidence of discussed or defined goals were observed. Physical care was considered by the raters to be acceptable, although some acts of physical care which were not acceptable were observed, but they reported that it was obvious that 'there was little evidence of insight into deeper problems and needs of the patient'(Wainwright and Burnip, 1983).

Summary

This part of the study was aimed basically at collecting base-line data to be used as feedback to the staff in the next phase and to be compared with later data. It took place before I joined the unit and therefore I had no influence or interaction with the staff at Burford.

The results suggested that the hospital staff held fairly traditional perspectives about nurses and their role and that the standard of care was average, or slightly less than that. The consumer population also held similar views of nursing to those surveyed in other studies. Burford Hospital itself was well liked by both staff and consumers, although a number of deficiencies were pointed out by both groups which suggested potential for change or development.

As well as being used later in the project, the data gave me an introductory understanding of the hospital, its staff and the people it served.

QUALITATIVE DATA

The second half of phase 1 began when I commenced as nursing officer at Burford Hospital. It involved a settling in and orientation period both of myself to the hospital, and between the staff, the community and myself. Overlapping with this time of orientation was the collection of subjective, descriptive data concerning the nursing work as well as a period of planned education. This stage continued for nine months, and ended when the nursing team as a whole agreed on the diagnosed problems to be subjected to planned change.

THE ROLE OF THE RESEARCHER

Until the beginning of this phase, I had had little contact with Burford Hospital. Commencement of employment as leader of this hospital demanded an examination of the amalgamation of roles in order to pursue the study.

I was employed as the unit nursing officer responsible for the nursing service in the hospital, and reporting to the senior nursing officer, who was not based on site. The Report of the Committee on Nursing (HMSO, 1971) suggested a hierarchial, supervisory structure for nursing, based on the industrial, scientific management model which emphasises clearly defined roles, with a line management structure to facilitate supervision (Davies, 1977). This was implemented throughout the National Health Service in the 1970s with the creation of Regional, Area and District Health Authorities giving a framework for the setting up of a nursing hierarchy. Burford Hospital was situated in a single area authority, that of Oxfordshire.

The role of the nursing officer, detailed in a written job description (Appendix IX), was that of both clinical nurse and nurse manager. The nursing officer was responsible to the senior nursing officer for the sector, who, in turn, was responsible to the divisional nursing officer, who was managed by the area nursing officer. Burford Hospital was one of four within the remit of the senior nursing officer, and a total of eleven hospitals, plus all district nursing, health visiting and other community services within the area were under the control of the divisional nursing officer.

Because Burford Hospital was small and geographically isolated, the nursing officer was also the senior officer of the Authority actually on-site. I was, therefore, responsible for the supervision and rostering of domestic, catering and other staff on a day-to-day basis, reporting to their appropriate departmental supervisors who were based off-site. Because of this somewhat broad brief, the nursing officer role was perceived to be one of overall leadership and of a figurehead by the nursing and ancillary staff; the paramedical staff; the medical staff; and, to a lesser extent, the community as a whole. The study demanded that I meet these expectations of the staff, the organisation and the community, while both attempting to change expectations and describe and evaluate the process.

I was to act as change agent alongside the adoption of the leader's role in the hospital, supported by the organisational, legitimate authority invested in it. Beckhard (1969) suggests that change agents are external − that is, from outside the organisation − and Archer *et al.* (1984) see them as being external consultants without legitimate authority. Mauksch and Miller (1981) argue that this is not necessarily required, but suggest that change agents employed within the organisation are a valid way of promoting change. Such 'internal' change agents must, however, be conferred with that specific role, and be officially designated as agents for change. Ottaway's (1980) taxonomy of change agents differentiates between those who promote and implement a change and those who adopt it, arguing that adopters are by definition inside the organisation. Promoters and implementors are portrayed as being from outside the organisation or employed by it specifically to bring about change.

In this study, the organisational head of the hospital was to become a truly internal change generator, implementor and prototypical adopter, a concept not discovered in the literature on change in organisations. Furthermore, the official *leader* was not only to be the official *change agent*, but also to act as a *researcher*. While Reason and Rowan (1981) strongly assert that the researcher of a social reality should become a part of the field setting and 'do' research with people rather than on people, and the qualitative school urges researchers to become immersed in the reality of the field as participant (Glaser and Strauss, 1970), the majority of studies based on such methodologies are reported from a stance where the researcher, although a participant, remains identifiable as a researcher only. Baker (1978), in her study of the attitudes of nurses to the elderly, which is based on participant observation, reports that those she participated with were told that she was a researcher, and that although she became 'one of them', this was only partly so because her boss wasn't theirs; her paymaster wasn't theirs; and she was there with an end in view, and a product of hers was in the making. Melia (1981), Glaser and Strauss (1970) and other authors of studies based on a grounded theory approach report on participant observation which was voluntary and a choice of method, rather than the author becoming organisationally participant. Action research studies, too, appear to be designed on the premise that the researcher is participant primarily as a change agent/researcher, and participation is a secondary role adopted as a means to collect 'real' data. James (1984), reporting on a period of participant observation with nurses (she herself being a qualified nurse), lists the comments of the other nurses she worked with, such as:

> 'Nicky, you're sort of like a p.s. in a letter. Not part of the main body of the nursing team, but still important.'

> 'This is our pet sociologist who's working on the unit and studying us. She's found out all sorts of interesting things.'

Although she, through participant observation, was able to perceive the reality of the world through the eyes of the nurses with whom she worked with more authenticity than the objective non-participant quantitative researcher, the reality may not have been as completely real, because she was seen as being somewhat different from 'subjects' of the research. Commenting on James' report, Bell and Roberts (1984) point out that she was 'really working', that is, in the eyes of the nurses, because she physically worked full shifts, but add 'albeit for free'.

The amalgam of the tripartite role I adopted was a deliberate attempt to take on full membership of the corporate identity of the nursing team alongside change agency and investigation through research. However, it was acknowledged that the plan was likely to be difficult to maintain, and that the early part of the phase would need to be used to help me come to terms with the three-sided role, and to convey and explain it to the staff who were to become participants in the study, rather than its subjects. It was also essential that, from the beginning, a disciplined and organised approach to observation and recording should be established.

In non-participant observation where quantitative scales are used, Treece and Treece (1977) suggest that a high level of precision can be achieved if the observer is 'well trained', since judgement is kept to a minumum. Abdellah and Levine (1965) say that it is less easy for non-participant observers to be precise or valid when qualitative data are collected because they have to exert judgement while standing outside the phenomena being studied. Participant observation, Denzin (1970) argues, is a more suitable method of qualitatively exploring phenomena, but it is seen as complex and demanding because of the intrinsic bias of the observer, who is aware of it, and yet unsure how to overcome it (Hall, 1978). Shaffir *et al.* (1980) note how such observers 'always live, to some extent, with the disquieting notion that they are gathering the wrong data, and that they should be observing or asking questions about another event or practice instead of the present one'. Glaser and Strauss (1970) say that researchers who choose participant observation must put themselves in the situation, get involved, yet, at the same time, maintain 'informed detachment' by planning opportunities deliberately to withdraw, write up, and then reflect. They are expected to trust their own credible knowledge, which they have gained by 'personal experience and analysis ... in what they have studied and lived through. They are prepared to convey the credibility of their observations in the written report'. The research strategy which evolves from such arguments is therefore one that would support the notion that the roles of organisational head/change agent/researcher be invested in one person, and the development of this was to be firmly rooted in this part of the study.

THE BEGINNING PERIOD OF ORIENTATION

The procedure followed was for me to become part of the workforce, fulfilling where possible the existing role and expectations of the staff, and to record the subjective data acquired as participant. The data were analysed and inferences made to form the basis of an initial description of the nursing work at the end of the three months.

Procedure

I took part in the 'Orientation programme for new staff' organised by the senior nursing officer, and worked full-time as the nursing officer. In a series of formal meetings, and informal individual discussions with every member of the nursing, medical, ancillary and paramedical staff, it was explained that I wished to 'get to know' the place, fit in as a member of the team and to avoid any 'new brooms sweep clean' changes. It was mentioned, however, that the intention was eventually to democratically plan for change, and that I was interested in what was to happen and would therefore keep records as the basis for writing up an account of experiences at the hospital.

A daily dairy was written over a period of 30–60 minutes, usually at lunch-time, and entries made at the end of the day when necessary. Occasionally, an entry was made immediately after an observation if it was felt to be important.

Data recording

The data were first recorded in narrative form, and then inferences made. A space was left to allow for notes to be added retrospectively. A typical entry would read as follows:

2 November 1981
Worked female side this morning with ... Met SN1 and SN2 and EN for coffee. SN1 complained that there were no spare staff cups and she wasn't

going to drink out of a patient cup. Offered to wash a patient cup for her but said she couldn't drink out of one. SN2 agrees with her, and the EN says she isn't going to have drinks charge deducted in future if no staff cups.

SNs unhappy about Mr ... because the doctor [Dr B] moved noisy patients into main ward so that a friend of his could be admitted to the side ward. SN1 suggests that I see Dr B about it, but to be careful. He understands, when I explain, that the noisy patient should be in the side ward because he disturbs people at night, but says that the patient in the side ward wouldn't like being in with others − if I can persuade her, it's OK by him.

Inferences:
1. Patients are dirty and contaminate cups, rendering them unsuitable for staff use.
2 (a) The nurses are not willing to challenge the doctor, even if the argument is sound.
  (b) They seem to want to rely on me as troubleshooter, and would be disappointed if I didn't do so.
  (c) The doctor accepts my argument, but is not prepared to reverse the decision himself − I as nurse can alter decision and face opposition.

Data analysis

The data from the diary were analysed manually, and categories created from the data, in order to describe what was observed. This was carried out by recording each observation point, and its associated inference, onto a 3×6 inch card. The cards were then grouped together according to similarities perceived, and each group given a categorisation label. Conclusions about the work and the hospital were then drawn from the inferences.

The following categories were used to sort out the 240 observation points and corresponding inferences that had been collected:

1. Organising and delivering care.
2. Patients.
3. Planning and recording care.
4. The multidisciplinary team:
    (a) The 'outside staff;
    (b) The 'inside' staff.
5. Role of the nurse.
6. Goals of the hospital/goals of nursing.

ORGANISING AND DELIVERING CARE

The daily work centred on the nine-bed ward, although other work impinged on this throughout the day. The minor casualty department was open twenty-four hours a day, and whenever someone came into the hospital for treatment a nurse from the ward had to respond to the bell, see the patient, contact the doctor and assist him when he arrived. This department also housed a doctor's clinic every Tuesday, Wednesday and Thursday morning, and a nurse was withdrawn from the ward to conduct these clinics with the doctor. Three to six elderly people were brought into the ward for the day at about 9.30 am, most of whom needed to be bathed, have dressings changed, and various other treatments.

The work flowed smoothly along a highly developed routine, with the day staff of two to three registered or enrolled nurses and two to three domestics beginning work at 8.00 am. The nurses began the day by listening, over a cup of tea, to the report of the night nurse in the ward office. The domestics remained in the ward during the reading of the report.

The reporting sessions consisted of a comment on each patient, and the following extract from the diary represents a fairly typical night report:

Night nurse (NN):	Right. Should I start?
Staff nurse (SN):	Yeah, let's have it them.
NN:	Mrs A had a good night. She had her sleeping tablets and slept all night. Mrs B says that she hasn't slept all night, but she was flat out every time I went round. Mind you, I wouldn't have slept all night with the noise Mr A's made all night. He's really getting worse. Spilt his bottle twice, and I told him in no uncertain terms not to try and do it himself, but he wasn't having any. Anyway, Mrs C's just the same and had her usual night. Now, Mr A. As I say, he's been terrible and been on the go all night, shouting for [his wife]. Spilt his bottle at 1 and 5. The largactil hasn't touched, and he's still wide awake now.
SN:	How much is he on now?
NN:	25 mg, but it doesn't touch him.
SN:	I know — but try and get Dr B to change it — you know what he's like.
NN:	Anyway, that's the family, and good luck to you, I'm off to bed.

The staff nurses then decided who would work where: a nurse and a domestic at one end of the ward area, a nurse and a domestic at the other. Another nurse would be allocated to cover the casualty clinic, and if another domestic were on duty, she would be expected to help out anywhere.

The whole team would then enter the ward area, and get the patients up, bathed and dressed. Dressings would be changed, and beds made, with the intention of having this all done before 9.30 am, when the day-patients were to arrive. At 9 am all of the nurses routinely went to coffee in a room just off the ward area. The domestics carried on with patients and bedmaking during the nurses' coffee break. At 9.30 am, the nurses' break ended, and the domestics, cook and porter took theirs. By this stage in the morning, all of the ward work needed to be complete, because one nurse would be in casualty at 9 am, and the day-patients would arrive at 9.30 am. At 10 am, baths for the day-patients would be carried out, with one nurse taking patients to one bathroom, and another to the second bathroom. The domestics would give assistance. A nurse would be left free to answer the telephone, and conduct the doctors' ward rounds. This would be the nurse who was seen to be 'in charge' – either the nursing officer or the full-time staff nurse. Most of the work finished, the staff normally congregated in the kitchen by 11.30 am for a cup of tea before 'dinners'.

At midday, half of the nurses would be sent for lunch, if the clinic was finished, and dinners would be served. Patients ate in bed or from tables in front of their armchairs in the sitting room. Medicines would then be distributed from the drug cupboard in the dressing room by two nurses, and all patients would be helped onto their beds for an afternoon rest. At 1 pm, the other nurses would be sent for lunch, and those left would write up notes in the office. Part-time nurses ended their shift at 2 pm, and one nurse would begin the 2 pm – 9 pm shift. Between 2 and 5 pm, two nurses and one domestic would walk patients back to the sitting room, serve tea at about 3 pm and begin to undress the patients at about 4.30 pm, helping them into their nightclothes. At 5 pm, the nurse in charge would read the day report, in a similar fashion to that of the night report, and the evening domestic would arrive on duty, leaving her and one nurse until 9 pm. Half of the patients would be put to bed before supper at 6 pm (cooked by the domestic) and the rest after supper. Lights were turned out between 7 and 8 pm, depending on how many needed help to get into bed, and the number of 'interruptions' by casualties, and the report given to the staff nurse and nursing auxiliary for night duty at 9 pm. Although all patients were now in bed, and the lights had been dimmed for some time, the first task of the night nurses was to prepare and give out milk drinks, and then to distribute night sedations and medications. After these rounds, individual calls were answered throughout the night; a number of regular cleaning and tidying jobs were carried out; and the night report written. At 6 am, lights were turned on and all the patients were given a wash and a cup of tea. The night nurses served breakfast at 7.30 am, which was cooked by the cook who began at 7.30 am, and the night report given.

PATIENTS

Thirty-one patients were admitted over the three-month period, and of these, 29 (93.5 per cent) were over the age of 65, and 27 (87 per cent), over 75. Three of these were transferred from the Oxfordshire District General Hospital following surgery, one having a removal of cataracts, one sustaining a broken wrist (colles fracture) and the other an abdo-perineal resection and formation of stoma. The other patients were admitted by their own doctor to give a 'break' for caring relatives (45 per cent, n = 14); with an acute illness such as stroke, pneumonia and unstable diabetes (26 per cent, n = 8); and for 'social reasons' when they were unable to look after themselves and needed care and rehabilitation (20 per cent, n = 6).

Patients for admission from the District General Hospital were initially referred to the nursing officer, who then had to contact a doctor to seek permission before accepting the referral if a bed was available. Patients admitted from home were arranged by the doctor concerned, who telephoned or called into the hospital, and told the nursing officer that the patient was to be admitted, gave instructions and any relevant information. Discharge of any patient was the prerogative of the doctor.

Since the average length of stay was 21 days, the patient population changed slowly — three patients remained in the ward for the whole of the three-month period.

Mrs A was a 67-year-old woman and was dying of cancer. She was weak, withdrawn and despondent, and required help with all of the physical acts of living, apart from feeding herself. Her daughter visited each evening. Mrs A sat out of bed for about one hour each morning and spent the rest of the day and night in bed.

Mr B was a 74-year-old man who was depressed, and who had been in the hospital on a number of occasions. He was able to get up, dress and walk with a frame unaided, although he did this very slowly and was often reluctant to carry out these activities without help. He needed help to get in and out of the bath. As in previous admissions, Mr B had neglected himself while at home (he lived alone in an old person's flat), and was admitted to hospital to be cared for, encouraged to eat a better diet, and to reduce his level of depression. In the past, a spell in the hospital had achieved a notable improvement, but he tended to deteriorate within a few months of returning home.

Mr C was an 84-year-old man who had suffered a stroke five months previously, and had been in the hospital since then. He was paralysed down the left side, and although he could feed himself and communicate well, he could do little else. A heavy man, two nurses were needed to lift him and dress him, and he spent most of the day in a geriatric chair, which tipped back and prevented him from slipping down. Mr C frequently became very distressed about his dependence, and wanted to do more for himself. For example, he did not like the nurses to help with positioning the urinal, and tried to do it himself, which often resulted in accidental spillages. He also attempted to stand from the chair on a number of occasions because he felt that he would be able to go home to be with his wife if he could walk. Because this led to a fall on two occasions, a fixed table, screwed across the chair, was kept in position to prevent him from attempting to stand. This was a source of much irritation to Mr C, who sometimes became angry when requests for it to be moved were refused, and he would respond by shouting for his wife, swearing at the nurses and banging the chair-table.

Patients liked the hospital, apart from Mr C, who thought some of the nurses were uncaring, although he spoke highly of others. As reflected in the consumer survey, local people felt a great loyalty to 'their' hospital, and the patients and their visitors mirrored this attitude, with frequent positive remarks to staff, expressions of thanks, and in their general behaviour within the hospital. They liked the 'feel' of the building, the 'friendly atmosphere' and 'being looked after by my own doctor'. There was no indication of dissatisfaction with the service or at having to conform to the routine, although some smilingly rationalized about the need for rigid routine:

'I'm in your hands. I don't mind what you and the doctor tells me, because I know it will help me to get better.'

'It is a bit like being in the army. But I liked the army, and you've got to have discipline if the work's to be done.'

'The nurses are so busy. They have to have set times or they'd never get done.'

Although one patient disliked being woken at 6 am, he felt that it was not unreasonable to be expected to do so, adding that 'they have a job to do'. Patients conformed to the 'rules' of the hospital with little complaint, and appeared to be very grateful for all that the nurses did. Even more gratitude was expressed towards the medical staff, whom the patients liked to see as often as possible and to whom all questions about progress, possibility of discharge and everyday matters of living were addressed.

Patient: I'm going to ask Dr D if I can start and get into the bath
           today. *to Dr D* I'm glad I caught you, because I wanted to
           ask you about my bowels. I haven't moved them for three
           days.
Dr D: Has the nurse given you anything?
Patient: Well, she wanted to give me some prunes for breakfast, but
           I said that I wanted to ask you about it first. *to nurse* Can
           you ask the doctor about Sarah [3-year-old grandchild]
           being allowed in?
Nurse: Oh, I don't need to ask the doctor, I can give permission
           for that — yes, that's OK.
Patient: I know you can dear, but I don't want to take advantage
           and I'd feel better if I could mention it to the doctor
           first.

While they 'appreciated' the care given by the nurses, they clearly felt
that they were 'ill people' who were in hospital to get better. The
doctor had arranged their admission, was treating their illnesses, and
the staff were there to carry out the plans prescribed by the doctor
when he wasn't there.

The nurses held a different view of the patients. Only two nurses
reflected in their behaviour that patients were ill and were in hospital
to get better. The others consistently asserted that the hospital should
only admit patients who were ill, and who would get 'better', or die
comfortably, and that most of the patients admitted should not have
been, because they 'were not ill':

'It's all geriatrics who should be in a geriatric home.'

'We get the odd interesting patient from the District General, but usually
it's just nursing old people with social problems who don't need much
nursing.'

'I didn't train three years to do this — anybody could look after
incontinent, old people.'

'I work here becuase it's convenient, but I'd love to do some proper
nursing now and again. I really miss it.'

'We're not nurses — shit-shovellers, more like.'

'They don't care what you do, as long as they are fed, watered, and clean:
well, forget about the clean bit, 'cos a lot of them don't even care about
that.'

'What rubbish have we got in now, then? [Nurse returning from holiday
at the beginning of morning report.]

All of these comments were made away from the patients' hearing. Most nurses behaved in a kindly, though detached, way with patients:

(*Two nurses approaching distressed male patient*):

Now, Mr E, what's the noise all about?

Patient: I've spilt the bottle. I'm sorry, nurse. (*He cries and puts hands over face*)

Nurse 1:   It's all right, Mr E — we'll clean up after you and you'll feel better. You should call us, you know, we don't mind helping you with the bottle. (*Patient continues crying and doesn't answer.*)

Nurse 2:   We'll go and get some clean linen, then sort you out, OK? (*Patient still cries with hands over face.*)

Nurse 2:   OK ... OK. Mr E? (*Patient nods his head, nurse leaves to go to the sluice room.*)

Nurse 1:   Oh God! I can't stand it — the awkward old bugger does it on purpose, you know.

Nurse 2:   He makes me sick.

Confused patients were less likely to get public kindness if they were disliked by nurse:

Patient: (*who was unaware of where she was*) What time's the bus due, dear?

Nurse: What bus?

Patient: The one to West Hanney. Mother will be annoyed if I'm much later getting home.

Nurse: Don't be stupid — your mother died years ago — you're 87, so she would be about 120 if she was still alive. There's no bus, so stop being silly.

Well-liked patients who were muddled were fussed over, however, and humoured. The following occurred in the sitting room immediately after the exchange above. Five patients were in the sitting room, and the two nurses were brushing the hair of a small, elderly, confused lady opposite the patient who asked about the bus. One nurse tied a red ribbon in the patient's hair:

Nurse 1:   There you are, dear — you look lovely, the men'll be after you, so be careful.

Nurse 2:   Doesn't she look sweet — you look lovely, gran!

Patient: She dropped it and broke it three times, exactly into three pieces.

Nurse 1:   (*kneeling down to position face level with patient's*) Who did what, love?

Patient: (*smiling conspiratorily*) You know who – you know –
             but I didn't tell anybody else who it was – three pieces, all
             smooth, as well you know.
Nurse 1:   Well, maybe we could fix it if it's smooth – were the
             pieces big or small?
Patient: It's in the bin – the men have got it – and nobody knows.
Nurse 1:   Well, that's all right then – don't you worry about it,
             love. You didn't break it and nobody knows anyway.
             (*Patient giggles and grasps nurse's hand. Nurse bends over
             patient, puts arm round her.*) Ooh, you're lovely (*looking
             at other nurse*) I could take her home and keep her.
Nurse 2:   Isn't she lovely?

PLANNING AND RECORDING PATIENT CARE

All patients were assigned a set of case notes for the use of the doctors
and paramedics, and a *Nursing Kardex*, stored in a visible register, on
admission. The *Nursing Kardex* had columns for nursing orders,
daily notes, and a frontsheet with spaces for basic biographical and
medical information. On admission, the nurse in charge at the time
would complete the biographical and medical section, and write an
admission entry. This entry usually consisted of a subjective
statement about the patient, such as 'nice old lady', or 'confused, but
co-operative lady'; the source and reason for admission, such as
'Admitted by Dr A following a fall at home, for observation'; and a
brief outline of care to be given, such as 'for bed rest, up to toilet,
4-hourly pressure area care. Drugs as per chart'. Occasionally, other
information was recorded such as 'uses false teeth', or 'unable to feed
herself' and specific medical information about diet, mobility, etc., if
mentioned by the doctor. Changes in the care were recorded in the
ongoing notes. Analysis of the nursing notes elicited little reference to
psychosocial care, except for family information if the doctor had
suggested that a social problem might exist.

THE MULTIDISCIPLINARY TEAM

The 'outside' staff

In addition to the nursing and ancillary staff, who worked together
and identified as one group, doctors and paramedics were employed
to serve the hospital. The nursing and ancillary staff frequently
referred to themselves as 'the hospital staff' who kept the hospital

running and gave a common-sense non-professional service, and saw the other members of the team as visiting experts who offered a knowledge-based, professional service. These feelings were not entirely favourable. The doctors, physiotherapist, social worker, district nurses and health visitor were all regarded as 'hit-and-run' practitioners, who came in, saw, issued orders and left the staff to act upon them. Observations in the diary reflect at least a daily reference to this situation by one of the nurses, for example:

> 'She wouldn't be so keen to order walking to the day room and back three times a day if she had to do it.'

> 'I wouldn't mind her job.'

> 'Mr F shouldn't be here. He needs good physio and Mrs G's only here what – no more than 3 hours a week on the ward.' – (These remarks refer to the work of the physiotherapist.)

> 'She says he isn't fit enough for part three. God, I wish I was clever enough to work that out from a five-minute chat in between filling in forms!'

> 'Margaret says that the family are really supportive, but he is really too heavy for them. He's not too heavy for us though – and she knows all about it, of course, because she's here so often, ha ha.' (These are references to the social worker.)

The most frequent remarks – made during tea-drinking, official breaks and report sessions – concerned the three doctors. The nurses regarded them with great ambivalence. On the one hand, they felt that the overall control by the doctor was legitimate, and they used the power of the doctor often to legitimate their own actions. Patients who did not want to get out of bed were told that the doctor said that they must (although no such instruction had been given) and this strategy was used to encourage conformity in patients to the routine for bathing, walking and resting on the bed after lunch. Conversely, decisions made by doctors were often the basis for heated discussion and criticism, although this was never raised with the doctors themselves. In particular, discharge decisions by doctors were rarely felt to be correct, with some patients being 'kept in' by the doctor when nurses felt they should go home, and some going home when the nurses felt they were not ready. Considerable anger was expressed about nurses having to set trays and then clear them when doctors wished to carry out procedures, especially if the nurse was not thanked. The nurses liked the doctors coming into the hospital, but they were uneasy about the feelings they experienced when they were there. 'There's been no doctor in this hospital for two days – the patients could all be dead as far as they know' was the general trend of a conversation at the nurses' coffee break at 9 am, yet at 11.30 am, the nurses commented on the doctor's visit at 10 am:

SN1:   What did he say about Mr H?

SN2:   He's taken the catheter out.

SN1:   I knew he'd do that. Did you ask him to come and change the wet beds, then? (*laughter*)

EN: Can you imagine him getting his hands dirty? Oh well, they don't realise, do they?

SN1:   I shouldn't have mentioned it really, I suppose. When he said 'catheter out', I thought, why can't he just leave it up to us? But they can't, can they?

SN2:   Did you tell him we had been washing it out with saline, and it was working?

SN1:   Yeah, he asked if I thought we should carry on with that, but I said I didn't know and what did he think?

RES: Well, what do you think would have happened if the doctor hadn't come in today?

SN1:   We would have got it running again with the washouts.

SN2:   We'd get on far better if they came when we asked them, instead of every day. You see, they interfere − I mean, to be helpful − but they do interfere.

SN1:   They are here far too often.

The doctors

The three doctors practising from the surgery in Burford had official admitting rights to the hospital, while neighbouring practices could admit with the permission of one of these three. No such admissions occurred in the three-month period.

In the Burford practice, the senior partner had been there for thirty-three years, and the two junior partners were his son and a friend with whom he had trained. Admissions to the hospital were arranged by the admitting doctor. All admissions were, therefore, controlled by the doctors. Discharge was also the prerogative of the doctor, who usually asked for opinions from the nursing officer.

Each weekday, one of the doctors would attend the hospital to conduct a ward round with the nursing officer, or the nurse in charge of the shift. The timing varied, but often coincided with lunchtime. The nurse would wheel a case-note trolley behind the doctor, who saw each patient, wrote notes at the bedside and wrote prescriptions. At weekends, doctors attended on request, although when the senior partner was on call, he tended to visit routinely. Discussions with doctors were almost entirely limited to myself, as nursing officer, or the nurse in charge of the shift. If I was on duty but busy, the doctor would usually wait until I was available to be on the ward round. The attitudes of the doctors were patriarchially benevolent. They supported the nurses and myself when criticisms from outside arose, and 'kept an eye' on us to make sure that we were 'managing'. Ownership of the patients was vested in the doctor. One doctor also made decisions on which specific bed was most appropriate for each patient, and spent much time in rearranging bed positions and furniture, and all of them made very basic decisions such as when patients could get out of bed and frequency of baths. Patients were classified according to the doctor. 'Whose patient is he?' meant 'Which doctor is responsible for this patient medically', and this question was asked frequently by nurses of each other. Doctors talked about 'my patients' at meetings, ward rounds, etc., and were quick to challenge any opinions expressed about patients from any member of the team which differed from their view, usually including in the retort that 'This is my patient and I am responsible for him/her.'

The physiotherapist
The physiotherapist worked three mornings a week and spent most of her time running an outpatient session in the physiotherapy room and seeing in-patients on the request of a doctor. She would usually carry out specific treatments with patients, only conferring with nurses if she wanted the patients to be walked in a specific way, or for a specified number of times each day by the nurses.

The social worker
The social worker covered three other hospitals, and called in at Burford Hospital once a fortnight on a fixed day, and organised a 'social work liaison meeting'. This was attended by the doctors, the health visitor, the district nurse and the nursing officer. Referrals were passed to the social worker at the meeting, who would see patients and report back to the doctors and nursing officer, informally or in a written report.

The health visitor
The health visitor was attached to the town practice, and was based at her own home. She was only seen at the hospital at the social work liaison meeting, and was responsible to a different branch of the nursing hierarchy – the nursing officer for health visiting, nine miles away.

The district nurses
District nursing needs were met by the team of district nurses based at the health centre of another practice 8 miles away. One nurse in the

team was designated to cover the practice patients, but she, as part of the other practice's team, relieved elsewhere and was relieved by a variety of nurses from the team. She, too, was only regularly seen in the hospital at the liaison meeting, but would occasionally call in to visit patients she knew, or when a request was made for her to continue care for a patient to be discharged home.

The liaison meeting

The liaison meeting was chaired by the social worker, and consisted largely of a dialogue between her and the doctors.

The 'inside' staff

The 'inside' staff were those who were exclusively employed for hospital work and consisted of:

Staff Nurse 1:   who worked full-time, and who had acted as nursing officer for eight months, between the previous nursing officer's retirement and my appointment.
Staff Nurse 2:   worked four days a week.
Staff Nurse 3:   worked three days a week.
Staff Nurse 4:   worked four days a week.
Staff Nurse 5:   worked four evenings a week.
Enrolled Nurse: worked full-time.

These nurses made up the day-shift nursing team. Also on the day-shift were a porter, who worked five mornings, a cook who worked five mornings, and seven domestics, who worked mornings and evenings. One of these domestics also cooked on two mornings, and all of them unofficially helped the nurses in addition to their domestic duties.

Four staff nurses and four nursing auxiliaries together provided night duty cover, with one staff nurse and one nursing auxiliary on duty throughout each night. I was the full-time nursing officer. The total nursing establishment was 9.5 whole-time equivalents.

The day nurses were regarded as the 'senior' members of staff and were expected to manage the care of patients according to the wishes of the nursing officer, who, in turn, was in full control of the 'housekeeping' aspects of the work, but in touch with the doctors who passed on their instructions about patient care.

The domestics, cook and porter were there to assist the nurses, were hierarchically below them and could be ordered to do tasks by them. If requests were ever perceived to be unfair, the nursing officer could be approached by anybody, although it was not 'good form' to report a nurse.

The night staff were a separate entity with little reference being made to them, although the nursing auxiliaries on night duties were perceived as nurses who did the same as the day domestics for more pay and with official acknowledgement of their role as a nurse.

The 'inside' staff identified strongly with Burford Hospital and were defensive of it. They had previously resisted suggestions, for example, to have volunteer programmes set up by the community because:

Staff: We don't want them in here – it causes more trouble than anything else, and too many things get out about the place.
Researcher: What sort of things?
Staff: Well, they whisper about people being made to get up, or being sedated or being made to eat and things.
Researcher: Being made to eat and things . . .?
Staff: Yes, you know, things they don't understand that there are good reasons for, and it gets the place a bad name, you know.

The world of patients and their community was seen to be different from that of the inside staff, and efforts were made to divide the two in the daily work. Patients and visitors were not to know that the staff drank tea or coffee when on duty; only titles were to be used to staff and not first names; there was a way to behave in front of patients; and a way to behave when apart from the patients:

(*Two nurses bed-bathing patient*)
Nurse 1:   I see you're still fag ashLil then? (*looking at ashtray on locker*)
Patient: Oh, yes, nurse. I've got to have me smokes.
Nurse 1:   It's not good for you, you know. Listen to your chest.
Patient: I know, but that's my only vice.
Nurse 1:   It's a filthy habit, though.
Nurse 2:   Look who's talking.
Nurse 1:   Have you had your son in yet? (*After leaving patient, in the coffee room*).
Nurse 1:   Don't let the patients know that I smoke – I felt really embarrassed.
Nurse 2:   I realised what I said as soon as I said it. She didn't notice.
Nurse 1:   Well, I changed the subject. She'll have to give them up though with that chest. I'll have another go at her after coffee.

The only behavour that was felt to be inconsistent with generally accepted 'good' staff behaviour and 'shown' to patients was that used to 'break the monotony'. The inside staff unanimously criticised the fact that all of the patients were old and that the work was monotonous. The way of coping with the monotony was, they voiced, to get on with each other and 'to have a laugh now and again'.

'You'd go mad if you didn't laugh.'

'We try and have a laugh and that keeps us going.'

'If you didn't laugh, you'd cry.'

None of the staff worked consistently in the ward for longer than two hours without some group withdrawal. Group breaks, official or unofficial, occurred with almost precise regularity at:

8 am
9–10 am
11.30 am
12–2 pm
3 pm
4.30 pm
6.30 pm
8 pm

At these times, staff would either meet in the staff room (if it was an official break) or in the wash-up area of the kitchen. No matter how 'busy' staff said they were, these periods were rarely missed, unless a doctor or a member of the nursing hierarchy was in the hospital, so they were aware that these withdrawals were not quite legitimate and must not be made known to people in authority. In the first two weeks of my orientation period, cups were hidden and cigarettes thrown down the sink by some staff when I appeared. This ceased quite rapidly when I accepted offers of a cup of tea and joined in.

Spontaneous 'fun' was generated throughout the day when it was accepted that I would not respond with a rebuke. Nurses filled colleagues' handbags with bandages, sanitary towels and assorted rubbish; the group would gather a member of the staff, cover her hair with talcum powder, spray her with air freshener or a syringe full of water, or put her fully clothed into a cold bath; cars would be draped with toilet paper; spoof telephone calls would be made to the hospital via the patients' trolley phone. Such activities occurred both away from the ward and in the ward itself. In the latter case, patients tolerated the noise – some joined in the laughter, others embarrassingly tried to avoid the antics by pretending to read or look out of the window. Again none of this took place when members of the 'outside' staff were in the building. On days when 'fun' did not occur, staff would remark on the day being dull or boring.

The frequent withdrawals and 'fun' appeared to draw the staff together into a unified group, to give them the strength to enter the ward and touch, talk to and look at the patients.

The link between the inside and outside staff was the position of nursing officer, which was seen as belonging to both, but really being on the side of the inside staff. Staff expectations of the nursing officer role were based on their experiences of the previous nursing officer, and the information given to them by the senior nursing officer that the new incumbent was an 'academic nurse' who was going to introduce changes and do some research.

The previous nursing officer was the subject of frequent discussion by all of the inside staff:

'Can you imagine what Matron would have said?'

'With Matron we couldn't ...'

She had been disliked by some of the staff (usually nurses) and extremely well liked by others (mainly domestic and auxiliary staff). Refusing to adopt the title of 'nursing officer', she had insisted on being called 'Matron', and lived in the flat which comprised the first floor of the hospital. The matron was thus on call 24 hours a day, answering all telephone calls and conducting the doctors' rounds. Although her management style was autocratic, and 'discipline was strict', the previous regime was liked by the community and patients, and the ancillary staff:

'You knew exactly where you were with her, and exactly what had to be done, when and how.' (Domestic)

'She was the old-style matron, and woe betide you if you were caught drinking tea − but you could hear her creeping down the stairs and disappear quickly. Silly, really − but she meant well.' (Domestic)

Giving patient care was not a part of the matron's role, and she was seen as a supervisor to whom respect was to be shown. The nurses were, on the whole, disparaging about that regime:

'We were nothing − we did all the work, but couldn't make any decisions, answer the phone, or even speak to the doctor.'

'She had her good points and bad points, like everybody. The routine was well worked out, and she insisted that patients were called by their proper name, like Mrs Smith. The patients loved her. But she didn't do any nursing, and ruled with an iron rod.'

However, in the nine-month period between the matron's retirement and the appointment of the new nursing officer, the staff

nurse who 'acted up' had changed very little. She had adopted
autocracy and preserved the routine. While the nurse in charge of the
shift was allowed to answer the telephone and accompany the doctor,
other nurses on duty at the time were not expected to do so. The
explanation for this was that nothing should be changed until the new
incumbent arrived, and there were suspicions that the old regime
might be satisfactory to the new nursing officer. Although the
previous order was not the one the nurses would choose, they had no
suggestions about how it should be changed, other than in workload
patterns, such as the cessation of having day-patients to care for in the
ward, and the buying of new equipment. Furthermore, they were
angry when the traditional role of the head nurse was not fulfilled
when I became the nursing officer.

'I think you are getting too familiar with the staff – Matron never did and
that was how she kept discipline.'

'It seems wrong for you to be looking after the patients. That's what we
are here for, and you should just be seeing that we do it.'

'I do think the boss has got to show he's boss. Otherwise people take
advantage.'

In summary, the inside staff were uneasy:

- They didn't much like the work, or the type of patients they cared
  for.
- They resented the authority of the doctors.
- They were unhappy about the authoritarianism of the old order.
- Yet, they appeared to value the routine, the doctors' presence and
  an autocratic leader.

THE ROLE OF THE NURSE

All of the nurses were qualified, one having state enrolment and the
others state registration, and there were no other workers officially
designated to give nursing care. In theory, then, the role of the nurse
could have encompassed giving total nursing care to patients. There
was, however, a hierarchy of tasks in patient care, and care delivery
was task-oriented.

The registered nurse's role focused on identifying which tasks were
to be carried out over a span of duty, and arranging for them to be
done, either through others or by herself. The tasks to be performed
were determined by the routine, the medical prescription and the
orders of the nursing officer. Thus, registered nurses carried out
predetermined tasks. Although the job descriptions for the domestics

did not include tasks related to patient care, the reality was different. Domestics joined with nurses to get over the peak work-times, particularly between 8 and 9 am, when patients were got out of bed and beds were made, and continued working alongside them in giving care. Personal hygiene, food service and talking to patients were seen as a common area of work for all staff, and not necessarily nursing work. Giving medicines, doing dressings and procedures, and dealing with telephone calls and doctors was perceived as the core of the nursing role. The latter were, therefore, highly valued tasks, and the former the province of anyone. Nurses commented that the monotony of the work lay in the fact that most of it centred on giving assistance in the acts of living, whereas they gained more satisfaction from medically/cure/treatment-oriented work.

'Bathing, dressing people is really unskilled work, isn't it? And you don't need to be a state registered nurse to do that.'

'I don't mind doing the basic care, it's just that I get more satisfaction from doing things that are more skilful.'

Nurses tended to get through the basic care as quickly as possible, or to delegate it to the domestics or the enrolled nurse where possible. The enrolled nurse was seen as a different kind of nurse. She liked giving basic care, and was not 'allowed' to give medicines or 'be in charge'. Much of the bathing fell to her, with the help of a domestic.

12 midday: Worked in the traditional way this morning. Did own ward round, took report with others, and then answered phone, did doctor's round and helped out in ward. SN1 went into casualty, SN2 worked with Dom 1 and EN worked with Dom 2. Dom 3 concentrated on cleaning sluices, etc. All of the in-patients were finished and in day room by 9, with the exception of Mr J and Dom 3 was detailed to help Dom 2 with his bath when nurses went to coffee. After coffee, six day patients had arrived, and all needed bathing. EN and Dom 1 bathed all of them, and the other two domestics cleaned and answered buzzers, took patients to the toilet, etc. SN2 did two dressings with day patients, gave out medications and sorted out the drug cupboard. Tea break at 11.30, asked her if she'd had a good morning: she said it was really good − got the work finished early, and because there were enough on, she was able to do those things a trained nurse should do, and the basic care was given well because she could supervise the domestics and the enrolled nurse. 'Qualified nurses should be there to do the skilled jobs, observe and supervise, and have enough auxiliaries on to do the unskilled work.' The enrolled nurse said that she agreed, and that was why she liked giving basic care, which she thought was real nursing. She said that the only people called nurse in big hospitals were pupils, students and enrolled nurses, because state registered nurses were called 'staff' or 'sister'. Therefore, the only time state registered nurses were nurses was when they were training to be one. The staff nurse looked irritated at this point, and said it depended on what you mean by nursing. Professional nursing, she said, was linked with medicine and needed medical knowledge and being skilled in drug administration and technical procedures. Two sorts of nurses were needed – highly trained ones to supervise and give technical care, and people with common sense to give the basic care.

Inference: Medical/technical care is skilful and requires training. Basic care is unskilled and can be carried out by anyone with common sense and minimal training. (Transcript from diary.)

Twenty-six observation points suggest that this view was commonly held both by the nurses and the domestics.

As nursing was closely aligned to medicine, it depended on instructions from the doctor, and involved translating the doctor to the patient and ensuring patient compliance with the doctor's prescriptions. Nurses identified with the doctors, presenting a united front to the patient rather than identifying with the patient, even if this proved to be painful, as can be seen in the following example.

Mrs A was in hospital for terminal care and was becoming progressively weaker and enduring much pain with fortitude. On three mornings in succession she requested that she be allowed to stay in bed, instead of spending an hour in the chair, because it was uncomfortable for her. The nurses refused the request each day, saying that the doctor had ordered that she be got up. On the third day, the doctor came before Mrs A was out of bed, and was asked if she could be left in bed. He felt that Mrs A was 'giving up' and should be made to get out of bed still. Staying in bed (for 24 hours instead of 23!) increased the risk of pressure sores. Despite the fact that the doctor did not see the patient, and the nurses were not invited to give an opinion, one nurse told Mrs A that she had asked the doctor about letting her stay in bed, and he had said no. Talking together later the nurses felt the decision was cruel, but preferred to comply with the doctor rather than the patient.

The role of the nurse was therefore predominantly perceived as one of operationalising the medical regime and carrying out technical tasks, managing and supervising care, and only giving care if there was no one else to do so.

THE GOALS OF NURSING

Nurses felt that they had achieved something if the work was finished on time or early; if patients got better; and patients looked comfortable and 'cared for'. 'Getting the work done' was the overriding goal on each shift, with frequent enquiries to each other about progress with work.

'How many beds left to do?

'How are you doing with the baths?

'Have you many patients left to do?

Staff in general became anxious if beds were not finished before 10 am, and a sign of a bad morning would be failure to do so:

'What a morning! We didn't finish the beds till half past eleven!'

Similarly, the end of each shift signified a stage of the work being completed. At 5 pm, patients should have been undressed and a half of them in bed; at 9 pm, all patients should have been in bed and the ward quiet, with the lights out; at 8 am, patients should have been washed, breakfasted, and the ward tidy; and at 2 pm, patients should have had a rest on the bed. Failure to meet such deadlines was translated as being failure to reach essential goals. When a nurse handed over at a shift change and admitted that the work goal had not been achieved, it was usually made clear that the nurses coming on duty were unhappy:

Day Nurse: Mr B is still up because he wanted to watch the news. I didn't think you'd mind, we've had a hectic evening with three casualties in.

Night Nurse: Is there anybody else to go to bed then?

Day Nurse: Only Mrs K − but she always stays up, doesn't she?

Night Nurse: Yes, usually, I just thought you might have put her to bed in place of Mr B. (*to nursing auxiliary*) You'd better put the milk on snappily or we'll never get them settled till midnight.'

Day Nurse: Look, I'm sorry, I just thought it would be nice for him to watch the news when he asked specially.

Night Nurse: Oh, it's OK, Sue, we'll manage − it's pretty quiet in the ward anyway.

Patients were required to look comfortable, and were directed by the nurses on what was and what was not comfortable:

(*Patient in day room has just pulled cushion out from back and put behind her head. The nurse walks in*)

Nurse: Oh, you look really uncomfortable, Mr D. Here, let me sort
          out that cushion.
Mr D: I've just put it there, nurse, it feels all right to me.
Nurse: I'll have it right in a jiffy, sit forward! (*Nurse puts cushion
          where it was before patient moved it*)
          There we are! That's better, isn't it?
Mr D: Thank you, nurse.

Two visitors have arrived to see a patient who is in bed − the nurses
walk into the room to check that the patient is awake. The patient in
the next bed has removed her pillows from the head of the bed and
laid them at her feet, and is fast asleep. The nurse places the pillows
back under the patient's head, waking her in the process, straightens
the counterpane and steps back and checks with her eyes for tidiness:
it appears to be tidy now, and she walks out and shows in the other
patient's visitors.

'Curing' patients with acute illness was a source of great
satisfaction to the nurses, with many recollections of those patients
from the past who were admitted very ill, and went home totally
recovered. Convalescent care of post-operative patients was also
gratifying to the staff:

> 'Three discharges this week − all good stuff. Anybody would think this
> was a hospital.'

> 'I feel as if we've really achieved something with Mrs E. A few more
> challenges like her would compensate for the other lot.' (About a patient
> admitted unconscious who recovered after three days.)

Patients who were not likely to be 'cured' were seen as the burden
to be borne, and patients who required active rehabilitation were
encouraged to be dependent to save time.

Mr A, one of the three patients who remained in the hospital for the
whole three months, was the topic of many conversations by the staff,
appearing in many diary entries. He was very unpopular with the staff
because he had been in five months at the beginning of the
observations and was heavy and 'demanding'. Left-sided paralysis
made it impossible for him to carry out all but the simplest self-care
acts, and he resented this dependence on others and longed to go
home to his eighty-year-old wife. Any possibility of that was not
considered by the hospital staff.

In the fourth week of the observation, I completed an assessment of
Mr A's self-care deficits, and a list of the basic movements which Mr
A would need to be able to master if he was ever to go home. Getting
out and into bed could be carried out by the district nurse, and a
regular bath could be provided as a day-patient. He would need to be

able to get from a chair to commode and back with the help of his elderly wife, and this alone was all that held him back from discharge. For two months, Mr A had worn a leg calliper during the day, and he had been 'walked' from the sitting room to the ward door and back three times a day by two nurses. This walking consisted of the nurses virtually carrying him, and one nurse pushing the foot of his paralysed limb forward with her own foot at each step. After six months in the hospital, it seemed that he was unlikely to be able to walk again. With the help of the physiotherapist, Mr A was taught to place his right hand on the high end of his bed, and pull himself up to a standing position, when one person would then place the paralysed hand in a grip over the bed end. It was then possible for one person to pull down his trousers, move the chairs from behind him, and replace it with a commode.

By the end of the three months' orientation period, plans were being made for Mr A to go home. The reactions of the staff to this were of excitement and success. Because he was seen as cured – although his basic condition was unchanged – he became popular and a source of pride. A transcript of a night report near the end of the three months contrasts with those typical of his earlier stay, such as the one reported earlier.

NN: Mr A slept for short periods. He was calling for his wife – I think he's really excited about going home.

SN: Mmm, isn't it marvellous! He's been here nearly eight months.

NN: Had a little accident with the bottle again – not incontinent – he just can't manage to move it from between his legs to the locker and doesn't think to ring for us. Can't we work out a way for him to do it?

SN: Yes, we'll have to think of something.

SUMMARY OF THE DATA ANALYSIS

All of the data-base derived from my subjective interpretation and was thus likely to be biased, given that much of the literature had been reviewed. Given that, Burford Hospital was found to conform with the findings of other studies and to reflect a style of nursing that change promoters in nursing assert to be the reasons why changes need to take place.

The work was highly routinised, based on the medical mode, and was pervaded with ambivalent attitudinal stances towards the old, the 'incurable' and about the role of the nurse in giving care.

The rigid routinisation of work is reported in many studies on nursing in all specialities, and the ambivalence towards care and cure has been identified in care settings where cure is not always possible, such as in psychiatry, young disabled units, mental handicaps and care of the elderly. Many of the conclusions of such studies were reflected in this study hospital.

Miller and Gwynne (1972) outline the range of attitudes which an institution may assume towards the care of patients – euthanasian, warehousing and horticultural. The euthanasian concept is the absence of any positive approach, and was seen with some patients at Burford. Warehousing is a system of segregation and paternalism, with the prolongation of physical value as the primary task. This approach conforms with Goffman's (1968) description of asylums as 'storage dumps for inmates'. Most patients at Burford Hospital, who were not suffering from a clearly defined acute medical problem, appeared to be subjected to the warehouse model, with its scrupulous attention to keeping things looking tidy and in order. Miller and Gwynne (1972) see it as the typical 'hospital' model concerned with people processing. When transferred to care achieving, the staff reinterpret care to mean the postponement of death for as long as possible, and patients are expected to be dependent. No different-iation is made between the care given and the need for it.

The horticultural model is one of development, with the encouragement of regaining capacities and attempts to reintegrate, or partially reintegrate, the patient with the outside world. The patient is viewed as having unrealised potential and is encouraged to become dependent. The staff are there to develop patients' abilities, not care for disabilities, and patients are more than the sum of the defective parts of their bodies. Little evidence of a belief in this approach was seen at Burford Hospital, although individual nurses sporadically adopted a similar approach with patients who were seen to be likely to be 'got home' if independence was encouraged.

An important component of Parsons (1951) sick role model is the demonstration of the motivation to co-operate in the treatment and return to normal. This is a prime element of the legitimate performances of the sick role. The old or potentially long-term patient may be seen as deviant (Field, 1972) through failure to improve or failure to co-operate. Furthermore, Field (1972) and Friedson (1975) suggest that such patients do not fit the medical model of cure and may not be liked by doctors. The historical dependence on doctors by the other staff may lead them to accept medical arguments, a feature of the work at Burford.

Although staff attitudes tended to favour the warehousing approach and the medical model, variations occurred with specific patients. Stockwell (1972), in her study of the 'unpopular patient', confirmed her suspicions that the patient's personal characteristics affected the attitude of nurses. Szasz and Hollender (1956) identify three models which are pursued in the doctor/patient relationship: activity – passivity; guidance – co-operation; and mutual participation. While guidance – co-operation is the most frequently developed doctor – patient relationship, the activity passivity approach is a feature of the nurse – patient relationship in the non-acute care settings studied by Miller and Gwynne (1972), and Goffman (1963, 1968), and was the norm at Burford Hospital.

The mutual participation model is seen as the most satisfactory in adult patient – doctor relationships, and is argued for in nursing by Murray (1976), Alfano (1971) and other nursing activists who advocate change. It is most likely to occur if the social distance between the two participants is minimal. Cartwright (1974) found that the middle class received more attention from doctors through the establishment of a peer relationship, and she also noted that those in higher socio-economic classes were to be found in the better equipped psychiatric and geriatric hospitals. Social distance is less likely to occur in the nurse – patient relationship because of the mix of socio-economic backgrounds of those who make up the nursing team. The nurse – patient relationship is often influenced by whether or not the patient is popular or unpopular, and this may be related to the personal characteristics of the patient rather than the social background. Stockwell (1972) discovered certain categories of patients were termed 'unpopular'. These included the demanding, the ill-humoured, the non-compliant and those with a physical deformity. The patients who did not distinguish themselves by extremes of behaviour were found, however, to be the most unpopular in terms of the time spent with them.

'Good' patients are those that cause the least trouble to staff, are quiet, clean and docile, and possess no physical deformity. Patient responses which are interpreted as 'awkwardness' were subjected to blunter and less sensitive handling.

'Getting through the work' appears to be a common phenomenon in giving nursing care. Clarke (1979a) found that ward staff were mainly concerned with the physical care of their charges and complained about anyone who stopped to talk to patients. On the geriatric wards observed in her study, staff worked under the strain of poor facilities and highly dependent patients, but were more satisfied than nurses on wards with less dependent patients, because the physical care to be given was obvious. Staff on the other wards were less satisfied because less dependence in patients meant, they said, they did not know what to do if patients did not need full physical care, and they could not identify their day-to-day aims. Differences between feelings of staff in non-acute wards and acute rehabilitation wards were also found by Coser (1964). Those who cared for less acute patients saw their roles as mainly custodial. They were concerned with cleanliness and neatness in the wards, were not concerned about patient activity, and saw themselves as separate from the patient. Those nurses in the rehabilitation oriented wards liked to see active, cheerful patients and saw the patient as an intrinsic part of their function.

This 'separative-ness' between the staff at Burford Hospital and the patients was a feature of the observation findings. Coser (1964) suggests that the nurse engaged in non-acute care is alienated from her work. She may find it meaningless, become estranged from the work situation, and isolated from other professional groups. The 'inside' staff at Burford Hospital were unhappy when 'outside' staff interfered in the work, but were equally unhappy if the 'outsiders', particularly doctors, did not visit. Work in long-stay and community or cottage hospitals does not bring professional recognition (Coser, 1964), and may be regarded as a 'step down' by other health workers.

Goffman (1963) describes the bi-cultural system which exists in care-giving institutions, with a patient culture, and a staff culture. Stannard (1973) discovered a sub-culture of behaviour within the staff culture. In many non-acute areas, untrained staff are employed in large numbers and Stannard describes how this leads to a polarisation of staff, with the untrained carers at one end of the axis and nurses at the other.

Among the untrained staff, the interpretation of patient responses is likely to be based on lay rather than medical ideology, because of their lack of knowledge. This leads to dependent people being controlled because they are 'like children'. Nurses respond from a medical perspective, and control is also legitimated because of the power of knowledge. Exerting control over patients becomes an appropriate belief within staff culture, although its legitimacy has a different basis according to the sub-culture. How control is exerted is seen as a problem by staff, and abuse may be accepted as a way to cope with it. A violation of the institutional expectations of proper patient behaviour may be seen as a 'punishable offence' and may provoke the staff not to give care, or give it in such a way that is unacceptable. Subtle verbal abuse and unfair responses to patients were apparent in this study. Dingwall and McIntosh (1979) comment that excellence is never achieved in respect of all patient care. Quality of care may be considered as a continuum, ranging from excellent, through acceptable, down to actual ill-treatment or cruelty. The lower end has received little attention in research studies, and Dingwall and McIntosh (1979) argue that too much attention in investigating nursing has been paid to the performance of tasks and single events, and too little of the everyday lives of patients and nurses. The Hospital Advisory Service (HMSO, 1971) report that little evidence of deliberate cruelty was found, but that a measure of neglect of patients was common.

Goffman (1963) argues that the system that is imposed by the staff culture is a means of controlling those who exist in the patient culture. Procedures are designed to minimise interference with staff routine and to maximise their convenience. Social distance between the two cultures is an integral part of Goffman's 'total institution', and it implies that the staff are in a superior position in relation to the patient. This distancing is maintained by avoiding the realisation of the patient's humanity, and by the staff agreeing that members of the patient group are different and inferior. The Burford Hospital staff repeatedly reinforced to each other the inferiority of the patients, concentrating on their being 'old' as well as on their dependence and 'being dirty'. Baker (1978) found that those nurses who were able to value the old patients they cared for were labelled as deviants, and could only survive through strength of character or in a team of nurses who collectively held positive views.

Coser (1964) says that members of staff who are absorbed into the staff culture and accept the system will become socialised into it, and those who object may leave because of the discrepancy between their professional self-image and what is actually going on. A third alternative is to withdraw as much as possible from the situation and leave the patient contact to the untrained staff. Davies (1976) suggests that nurses have taken on board handed-down, menial, medical tasks, and have hived off the basic tasks of nursing to the untrained. Many writers note how the bulk of care is given by untrained or student nurses, and that qualified nurses do not give patient care. The socialisation of nurse training indicates the belief that patient care is lower-order work, and technical procedures represent higher-order work. Miller and Gwynne (1972), in their study of long-term institutions, found that nurses were happy in giving medicines, injections and identifying illness, but not in giving care to the inmates. Total patient care is seen, however, to be extremely complex by Pembrey (1980) and the role of the nurse in the wards she studied where this was practised demanded high expertise. Menzies (1960) reports on the high anxiety inherent in being with patients. Hall et al. (1975) suggest that the untrained nurse cares for a patient in a way that merely 'safeguards and maintains' and is passive and static, whereas trained care-givers are capable of engaging in 'reversing a process, that is, bringing about an acceptable change in addition to safe-guarding', which is 'active and dynamic'. Despite such evidence, empirical descriptions of how nursing is given suggest that the delegation of patient care to untrained nurses as was the norm in the Burford Hospital, extends throughout the National Health Service.

The data and inferences from this first three months of phase 1 were collated, analysed and prepared for presentation in the next part of the phase. It was hoped that the information would give awareness to the hospital staff about their work, and of current knowledge about hospitals, patients and nurses as a prelude to identifying problems, or diagnoses, which could be concentrated on in the change process.

6 Burford as it could be

EDUCATING BURFORD

Having collected and analysed base-line data concerning Burford Hospital and its nursing work, the next step in the phase was to feed back this information to the staff, and to increase their knowledge base on contemporary ideas on nursing.

An educational programme was constructed around the findings and permission sought from the senior nursing officer to incur extra revenue costs by employing an extra nurse for three hours a week for six months. This was to allow for a weekly afternoon seminar. After considerable delay, this request was granted. Throughout the six months, I continued to be part of the workforce, led the seminar group and did not introduce any major practice changes other than those imposed by the organisation, or minor changes which were inevitable because of events. For example, a new medication administration system was introduced, using a lockable trolley which was wheeled around the ward, because the old procedure did not meet with organisational policy and the nursing hierarchy insisted on the change when that became known. Similarly, a full-time nurse was employed when one of the part-time nurses resigned, and a previously unfilled vacancy existed. The daily diary that I kept was maintained, and I made extended entries after the group sessions.

Staff development programme

Twenty-four seminars were planned, and a programme was presented for these to be held every Monday afternoon. All of the nurses were invited to attend, and it was explained individually to each nurse that the next six months were to be a time of thinking about the work in the hospital, learning about new ideas and deciding what needed changing.

75

Throughout the period, all of the day nurses attended each week, but the night nurses were unwilling to do so, and requested a 'special' session for themselves. It was agreed that a three-day workshop would be organised towards the end of the six-month programme, for the night staff.

THE SESSIONS

Table 6.1   Staff development programme, phase 1

Week	Session	Individual projects
1	Introduction, fieldwork feedback, discussion of planned programme	Guided reading
2	The patient – who is he or she?	Formulate own beliefs for presentation at session 3
3	(a) Discussion on 2 (b) What is nursing?	Guided reading
4	Nursing as it is now – comparing 3(b) with nursing at Burford	Guided reading
5, 6,		
7,	Models for practice	Guided reading
8	A model for us? Discussion on the relevence of models, etc.	Prepare discussion paper on own views
9	Presentation of individual discussion papers	
10, 11	Organising care	Guided reading
12 – 18	The nursing process	Guided reading
19 – 22	Role play – patient simulation	
23, 24	Identifying problems that need changes to overcome them	

Session one

The first session was a free discussion centred on the results of the previous data collection, and about the programme itself. It was a heated afternoon, with some of the staff feeling angry about my inferences, but I tried to explain that the purpose of the feeding back of the findings was to 'check out' their validity with the staff: 'Are the things I suggest only my opinion? They may well be, and only you as a group can explain the differences.'

It was agreed that the relevant parts of the findings would be related to each week's discussions so that, for example, the inferences and data from which they derived concerning the nurses' attitudes to patients would be discussed in weeks 19 – 22 alongside the lay teaching sessions about the nurse – patient relationship. Sessions 2 – 18 would consist of the presentation of a seminar paper by either myself or the group members, and then discussion of the paper by the group. Because the group members knew each other, and I was a working member of the team, discussion was always lively and easy. Relevant feedback from the preliminary fieldwork was included and the ideas discussed were related to Burford Hospital.

Session two

The second session asked the group to consider the nature of man, and argued that before nurses could be clear about who they were, what they should do and what their contribution to care could be, it was necessary to agree on a basic philosophy of nursing which encompassed beliefs about man (Mayers, 1972). Brief accounts of the theories and philosophies of Plato, Marx, Freud, Sartre, Skinner, Christianity and holism were given, and the concept of holism was explored in greater depth.

Mayers (1972) regards a 'well-defined philosophy as critical to a nursing agency. It determines the basic principles of care and the nursing relevance of the nursing methods that are employed'. Many nursing theorists, such as Orem (1980) and Roper *et al.* (1980), argue that nursing must view patients as holistic beings, basing nursing on a philosophy of man where 'the person is believed to be an integrated whole with biological, psychological, sociocultural, philosophical and intellectual components' (Sundeen *et al.* 1976).

The term 'holism' was first used by Smuts (1926) to describe his belief that the determining factors in nature are wholes. He says that it is a law of nature that living things are a coherent system constituting a complete group of sub-units that work together as one. The whole person is a system with sub-systems that operate as an entire unit. He or she is more than the sum of his or her parts, and the parts are mutually dependent and intrinsically and systematically co-ordinated. In nursing, the holistic view means that each client must be regarded as a whole person (Beyers and Phillips, 1971), and it is, according to Reihl and Roy (1980), becoming a widely accepted philosophical basis within circles of nursing leadership from which nurses can develop an understanding of what nursing is. This session's content was new to the group and was greeted with some controversy. Some participants identified with the need to begin with an understanding of the nature of man, while others suggested that it was merely an intellectualising of common sense.

Session three

The first part of the session considered the individual beliefs that each nurse had written down. All presented statements which reflected a belief in the worth of the individual, and the notion of holism, but it was difficult to ascertain how much of this was influenced by the growing loyalty of the group to me as a co-worker who could 'tell us about a lot of interesting things we've never heard about before'. This strong loyalty grew in strength as the other sessions proceeded, so that, as time progressed, much of the content of the seminar papers became a part of each nurse's belief system.

The seminar paper concentrated on attempts by nurses to define nursing. The most widely known definition is that of Henderson (1966):

> The unique function of the nurse is to assist the individual, sick or well, in the performance of those activities contributing to health or its recovery (or to a peaceful death) that he would perform unaided if he had the necessary strength, will or knowledge, and to do this in such a way as to help him gain independence as rapidly as possible.

Many other definitions have been suggested. Bower (1972) sees nursing as 'the application of knowledge to promote and maintain maximum health, comfort and care'. She also points out the uniqueness of nursing in its property of being able to operate in a highly generalised manner. Travelbee (1971) expands on this generalistic function and stresses the fact that the nurse is there with the patient twenty-four hours a day. Tiffany (1977) concurs with this emphasis, adding that nurses 'are present at the birth and death of most of us, and could be considered the worker bees of the system'.

The contemporary acceptance of a humanistic approach is reflected in most of the stated definitions, and nursing is often seen as an essentially social activity. As such, the importance of developing relationships – both between nurse and patient, and nurse and co-health workers – is often central. Chapman (1979) proposes that nursing is a 'social activity, an interactive process between individuals, the nurse and the patient', whilst Sundeen *et al.* (1976) see the nurse as 'being involved with all the components of a person in a dynamic interaction'. La Monica (1979) says that the goal of nursing is 'to provide humanistic care adapted to individual needs'. Thus, contemporary nursing theory asserts that nursing involves seeing the recipient as a holistic being, and using this view to meet his or her individual needs through meaningful interaction.

Discussion in this session took two lines. The nurses had not considered nursing in these outlined ways, and found it both illuminating and helpful. Much discussion led to an agreement with all that the theorists offered! It was felt, however, that these theories concerned how nursing should be, and that nursing within Burford Hospital fell far short of the 'grand' theories. The group felt that this state of affairs existed because, until this discussion, the nurses had never consciously thought about the nature of nursing, and saw it as a set of unrelated tasks, dependent on the medical diagnosis and prescription.

Session four

The discussion of the last session was developed, leading the group to suggest that nursing should be an interactive process, aimed at meeting individual needs, and, consequently based on the patient's individuality. The complexity and impracticality of defining nursing was discussed at great length, and I raised the notion of constructing conceptual models, rather than stating definitions.

Roper (1976) asserts that it is not possible to describe adequately what nursing is in a crisp, concise definition. She says that only a broad schematic explanation of an interpretation of what nursing someone entails, presented in the form of a conceptual model, can give meaning to the reality of nursing. Some nurses such as McFarlane (1976) reject any moves to impose rigid definitions of nursing on its practitioners. She further suggests that models are 'conceptual representations of reality', of use in developing nursing as a human service. Reilly (1975) argues that they are essential to give nurses 'a perspective, a way of looking at nursing'.

Sessions five to seven

The next three sessions proved to be very heavy going, and the group found much of the American literature confusing. After considering different nursing models, the group requested to pursue only one model in depth, chosing that model developed by British theorists (Roper *et al.,* 1980) as most appropriate to their work. McFarlane (1976) argues that all nurses should practise from a knowledge-base which is sufficient to enable her to justify the actions she takes, and that 'professional' nurses should base practice on a conceptual model. The discussion of developing nursing models is plagued with confusion in the literature. McFarlane (1976) comments on the 'utter semantic confusion' in theorising in nursing, suggesting that it is 'doubtful if clarity can be restored'. Citing Dickoff and James (1968), she observes that nursing grasps at 'concrete, structural security too soon', and asserts that 'like the world of the infant, the world of theory in nursing seems a "blooming, buzzing confusion"'.

Johns and Davis (1975) describes a conceptual model for nursing practice as a 'systematically constructed, scientifically based, and logically related set of concepts which identify the essential components of nursing practice together with the values required in their use by the practitioner'. This 'diagram', as it were, of what nursing is provides for the nurse a diagnostic and treatment orientation for the specific practice of nursing (Reihl and Roy, 1980). The 'diagnosis and treatment' refers to *nursing*, and not to the acts of medicine.

Reihl and Roy (1980) suggest that the current development of nursing models is a serious attempt to provide alternatives to the disease/medical/hospital-oriented models of the past, and say that contemporary nursing, for the sake of the patients, needs to develop models specific to nursing. In using the 'Nursing Process' as a means to deliver nursing care, nurses have need of a conceptual model on which to base assessment, identification of patient problems, planning care, implementing care and evaluation of outcomes.

Orem (1980) suggests that if nurses use the concepts and theories inherent in a model, they will practise more effectively, and will be able to 'place in perspective, other descriptions of nursing including those in other areas of specialisation'. Both she and Roper (1976) believe that a satisfactory model will describe nursing in any context, and will have meaning for nurses in all specialities. Orem (1980) goes on to observe that through the emergence of models specifically for nursing, the nurse's role is 'emerging from obscurity imposed by an over-emphasis on the relationship between the physician and the nurse, and between the employing institution and the nurse. . . . Nurses are coming to recognise that an item of information about a patient may have one meaning for a physician, but quite a different meaning for the nurse'.

A number of models are described in the literature, and an attempt is made by Reihl and Roy (1980) to construct a unified model for nursing by amalgamating a variety of models. In their classification of nursing models developed to date, they suggest that three types emerge: systems models; developmental models; and interactionist models.

In the first two sessions on models with the group, systems models were discussed. The basic premise of those nurses who favour a systems approach is the concept of an open system within an open system. Byrne and Thompson (1978) recommend that humans can be understood in the context of the subordinate system of which they are composed, such as cell, organ and organ systems, and the superordinate systems in which they exist − the family, the community and society. Systems theory uses a concept of man as an organism, existing in a steady state, being subjected to stress and then adapting or adjusting in order to re-establish its stability within the acceptable parameter. Orem (1980) and Roper *et al.* (1980) both place extra emphasis on development and interaction, and, although systems-based, expand the conceptualisation outside the narrower confines set by those theorists who pursue a purist systems approach. While the group preferred the model of Roper *et al.* (1980), they acknowledged conditional acceptance of Orem's self-care concept of nursing, but were irritated by the language and jargon used.

The other systems were dismissed as either meaningless, irrelevant, or 'a lot of hooey about nothing'! Those models discounted were those of Bower (1972), Saxton and Hyland (1975), Neuman (1980) and Roy (1980).

Roper (1976, 1979) and Roper *et al.* (1980, 1981, 1983) describe a model which incorporates many of the concepts implicit in the model described by Orem (1980) and the concept outlined by Henderson (1966). Roper's model for nursing is based on a model for living, and attempts to describe the reality of nursing to help nurses to develop a mode of thinking about nursing which focuses on the process of living. Developed from the findings of a research study into clinical experience of student nurses (Roper, 1976), the purpose of the model is to develop nursing as a discipline. Wilson (1972) purports that disciplines are 'forms of thought that have a characteristic approach to appropriate questions related to a subject'. Roper (1976) suggests that the use of a model will allow nurses to think 'nursologically', that is, in a way characteristic to nursing, in the same way that mathematicians think mathematically, theologians theologically, and anatomists anatomically. She asserts that her model is 'an attempt to initiate a conceptual structure for nursing which could be used as a base from which the discipline of nursing could develop'.

Roper *et al.*'s (1980) model for nursing identifies the subject of nursing as the individual, seeing him or her as a person engaged in living through his or her lifespan. Related to, but not entirely dependent on, the lifespan is a dependent – independent continuum, the individual moving towards each end of the continuum dynamically, depending upon the developmental stages of the lifespan, and immediate circumstances such as environment, state of health, etc. In living, the individual partakes of, or requires help with, four groups of activities, all four of which are interrelated, and are only divided into discrete entities for the purpose of analysis. The four groups of activities are:

1. activities of living;
2. preventing activities;
3. comforting activities;
4. seeking activities.

From these concepts, a model of living is constructed. Although all four groups of activities are so interrelated that, in reality, they cannot be seen to be separate, Roper *et al.* (1980) argue that discussion of them separately clarifies the nature of nursing.

ACTIVITIES OF LIVING (ALs)

Most people engage in the full range of these activities in their daily life. However, there are stages in the lifespan when the individual cannot yet, or no longer can, perform one or more of the activities, and specific circumstances may restrict performance in one or more activities. There are times in the lifespan when the individual is at a point nearer to the dependent or independent pole of the dependence – independence continuum and movement along it is dynamic.

Performance of the ALs involves the three other groups of activities, so that preventing, seeking and comforting activities are all involved with:

● Maintaining a safe environment
● Breathing
● Eliminating
● Controlling body temperature
● Working and playing
● Sleeping
● Communicating
● Eating and drinking
● Personal cleansing and dressing
● Expressing sexuality
● Dying

Preventing activities

These are the activities that individuals engage in to prevent those things, such as illness and accidents, that will impair living. They include a vast array of almost unconscious acts performed as a result of socialisation.

Comforting activities

These are the activities that a person performs to give physical, psychological and social comfort.

Seeking activities

These are the activities that the person engages in in the pursuit of knowledge, new experience and answers to novel problems.

Roper (1976) emphasises the closeness and overlapping of these four groups of activities. If a person is suffering from an extreme headache, he or she will, by carrying out certain ALs, *seek comfort* by consulting a doctor and thus try to overcome the complaint and *prevent* it from reoccurring. The model of living represents the individual − the subject of nursing − engaged in the process of living. Roper (1976) describes the subject of nursing thus:

> Basically, man is envisaged as carrying out various activities during a lifespan from conception to death. His main objective is to attain self-fulfilment and maximum independence in each activity of daily living within the limitation set by his particular circumstances. He also carries out many activities of a preventing, comforting and seeking nature and he appropriately alters priorities among the activities of living. In these ways, the individual endeavours to be healthy and independent in the process of living.

Roper *et al.* (1980) develop their model for nursing using the model for living. Illness is seen as but an episode in the life of an individual, and it is proposed that nursing must be approached within the context of the patient's process of living. Nursing is modelled as being composed of four components, which equate with the four groups of activities in the model of living.

AL COMPONENT OF NURSING

This is the central component of nursing, and is concerned with the acquiring, maintaining or restoring of maximum independence for the individual, or enabling him or her to cope with dependency in any of the ALs should that eventuate. Nursing may need to inform, counsel, provide material resources for, or actually carry out activities for, the individual.

Preventative Component of Nursing

This is essentially a part of every nursing activity. It includes the prevention of such things as pressure sores, dehydration, boredom, etc., as well as facilitating the acquisition of knowledge by the patient to prevent ill health. This component is modelled as supporting the AL component with the objective of minimising dependence.

Comforting component of nursing

This may be equated with the nurturing aspect of nursing, seen as fundamental to nursing (Hall, 1964) or the 'art of nursing' (Roper *et al.*, 1980). It includes such things as helping the patient into a position of physical comfort, taking a hand in an offer of companionship and placing needed items within easy reach. This component is inherent in every interaction between nurse and patient. It is modelled as supporting the AL component with the objective of maximising independence.

The dependent component of nursing

In the model of living, seeking activities are identified as one of the four groups of the dependent component of nursing aims at meeting the goals of these activities. When a person is ill, medical help is sought and nursing may be required. When a person is unable to reach maximum level of independence, although not ill, nursing may be needed without medical input. The dependent component of nursing exists when medical intervention is appropriate, and consists of tasks prescribed by a doctor, to be carried out by the nurse. The nurse is dependent upon medical prescription to fulfil this component of nursing, and it is not always an element of nursing for every patient.

To put this operationalising model into practice requires the use of the 'process of nursing' (Roper *et al.*, 1981). The model and the process can then be combined to construct an action model for nursing (Figure 6.1).

The Roper *et al.* (1980) model was unanimously welcomed by the group as a guide to their proposed 'new' practice norms. They felt that it well described what nursing could be; it was useful to explain clearly to non-nurses what nurses did, and they felt that they understood and identified with it fully.

Session nine

This was an open discussion based on individual papers presented by the group on nursing models. The overall feeling of the group was that using a model would clarify their thoughts; create a shared understanding of the nursing role in the study hospital; focus on patients rather than nurses; and give nurses more strength to delineate their contribution to care, in the multidisciplinary clinical team. They were extremely critical of all the US models, largely because they had difficulty in understanding the language used.

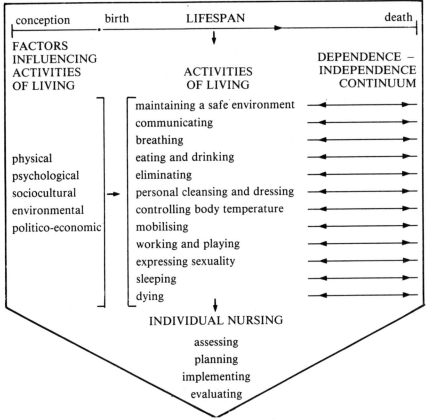

Fig. 6.1 Model for nursing

Sessions ten and eleven

These began with a discussion of how care was organised in the hospital, and consideration of task assignment, delegation of nursing to unqualified nurses and continuity of care. The seminar paper presented considered alternative methods of organisation.

Marram (1979) purports that any method of organising nursing should aim at:

1. Unifying the patient's care to minimise fragmentation.
2. Placing nursing care at the patient's side to avert the pyramiding of nursing care delivery and the nurses' preoccupation with hierarchy.

The methods of team nursing, unit assignment and primary nursing are all attempts to achieve such objectives.

TEAM NURSING

Kron (1976) maintains that team nursing is more a philosophy than a method of organising nursing; and Barrett (1968), while agreeing with this, suggests that it is also a methodology for delivery and organisation of nursing work:

> Team nursing is said to be a philosophy rather than a way of working. Perhaps it is both, for patients are assigned, and staff is organised in special ways when team nursing is practised. Yet as a philosophy, team nursing expresses beliefs about patients, personnel, leadership and relationships.

A team is a group of persons working together towards a common goal *(Kings English Dictionary,* 1930). A nursing team, according to Leino (1951), is a 'group of professional and non-professional nursing service personnel working together in planning, given, and evaluating patient-centred nursing care to a group of patients'.

Team nursing aims at achieving nursing care objectives through the action of a group of nurses, and is based on a belief that participative management gives better job satisfaction and motivation. The nursing team is composed of two or more members of staff (one being designated as leader), who are assigned the care of a group of patients. Advocates of this method state that the leader must be a registered nurse (Leino, 1951; Lambertson, 1953; Barrett, 1968; Kron, 1976). In a ward where the number of patients is small — Barrett (1968) suggests below fifteen — only one nursing team may be needed, but in larger wards, two or more team leaders and their teams may function under the direction of the ward sister. The team leader is delegated responsibility for providing care, and through a daily team conference, assigns individual members of the team to specific patients.

As a method of nursing care delivery, team nursing began to be used in Britain some years ago and was seen to offer a number of advantages. As the team assigned to care for the patient is constant, the patient is able to develop relationships more easily with carers, and continuity of care is promoted. As authority is decentralised, the team leader is given an opportunity for growth in terms of leadership skills, and supervision of untrained staff is closer. Manthey (1973) and Marram (1979), however, are critical of its capacity to facilitate individualised care. The method is often misinterpreted by clinical nurses and often leads to task assignment.

UNIT ASSIGNMENT

Sjoberg *et al.* (1971) describe a method of organising nursing based on the progressive patient care concept, and call it 'Unit assignment: a patient centred system'. Developed for a Canadian hospital setting, the method is based on findings from an extensive preliminary research study aimed at identifying the activity patterns of nurses involved in patient care, and establishing a method by which high-quality, patient-centred care could be provided within the existing constraints of staffing policies (Holmlund, 1967; Sjoberg *et al.,* 1968; Sjoberg and Bicknell, 1969). In line with the progressive patient care concepts, the method developed classifies patients into four care levels:

1. intense;
2. above average;
3. average;
4. minimal.

From this, Sjoberg *et al.* (1971) developed the unit assignment method, where the ward structure is decentralised, and divided into care units for each of the four care levels. Each small care unit is complete in terms of equipment and facilities, and the nurse's station for each is situated close to the patients. Each day, the patient's classification is reviewed and placed in the corresponding care unit.

Within each care unit, nursing is said to be patient-centred and the nursing team operates in the same way as that in team nursing.

Although unit assignment is an efficient way to utilise nursing staffing resources, critics such an Manthey (1973) suggest that it militates against the establishment of meaningful relationships between patients and nurses, and thus continuity of care. There is a possibility that the movement of the patient from one care unit to another may well give rise to anxiety or distress.

PRIMARY NURSING

Manthey (1970), describes this method of organising care where every patient is assigned a primary nurse who cares for him or her throughout the hospital stay when she is on duty, and care is delegated to a secondary or associate nurse when she is off-duty. Each primary nurse has a caseload of patients, and holds 24-hour, seven days a week responsibility for planning and administering care. The associate nurse follows the care plan developed by the primary nurse in reports by Hegyvary and Haussman (1976), but Manthey *et al.*

(1970) suggest that the associate 'may change parts of the care plan to reflect changes in the patient's condition; however, the primary nurse is responsible for any fundamental changes in the design of the plan'. Manthey *et al.* (1970) and Manthey (1973) relate the introduction of the primary nurse method in a medical ward. Each qualified nurse was given primary responsibility for a group of three to six patients and the skill of each nurse was considered in assigning her to patients. The primary nurse in this area assesses her/his patient on admission, prepares a plan of care with the patient, and is responsible for implementing the plan and its continuous evaluation. When off duty, they delegate responsibility to their associate. Primary nursing appears to have become well accepted, and is 'alive and well in the hospital' (Manthey, 1973). Christman (1973) describes how the large hospital he is associated with has introduced the method throughout all specialties and has recruited an all-registered nurse staff to do this.

Elpern (1977) criticises the approach on the grounds of poor feasibility, but agrees with the concept and describes 'modular nursing', which is a method that supports primary nursing. It is based on geographically defined care units in the ward, with 10–12 patients. Nurses are permanently assigned to the care unit or 'module', with off-duties arranged so that staff within the module cover others who are off-duty. The module leader has 24-hour responsibility (i.e. she is the primary nurse) and has the opportunity to move to all shifts, should she so wish.

Donovan (1971) suggests that the chosen method of organising care chosen is not important, as long as it is one that decentralises authority and focuses on the patient. The group were interested in the new methods discussed, and felt that task assignment was inappropriate. They decided, however, to reserve judgement in making decisions about a method until the planning phase.

Sessions twelve to eighteen

Six sessions were devoted to exploring the nursing process – a concept being widely advocated at the time in the nursing press and the subject of much discussion throughout nursing. The group had little understanding about the nursing process, and the sessions were very much didactic at first, until the group felt able to contribute.

Elhart *et al.* (1978) define the nursing process as 'the framework through which the nurse functions to meet specific responses in the provision of patient care'. Many authors base the process on the scientific, problem-solving process, which has been adapted to fit the activities of a number of occupations. De Cecco (1974), for example, in describing a teaching model compares it, and most other teaching models, with the problem-solving process.

Larkin and Becker (1977) suggest that without the ability to use problem-solving, nurses are 'forced to function by rote depending on memorised facts, and knowledge may be obsolete soon after a nurse graduates'. Johnson and Davis (1975) also see the skills involved in the nursing process as the same as those in problem-solving. They say that problem-solving is 'the key technique in the nursing process'. Sundeen *et al.* (1976), however, differentiate between the problem-solving process and the nursing process by saying that 'the problem-solving process is the development of new knowledge. The purpose of the nursing process is to maximise a client's positive interaction with his environment, his level of wellness and his degree of self-actualisation'.

Campbell (1978) sees the use of nursing process as 'the basis for professional practice which is flexible enough to serve as a skeleton for most nursing functions'.

The framework of a process gives steps through which to move. Roper *et al.* (1980, 1981, 1983) and Pearson and Vaughan (1984a) suggest the same four-step approach to the nursing process, which summarises these more lengthy plans of other writers:

1. Assessment,
2. Planning,
3. Implementing,
4. Evaluating.

Assessment includes data collection and identification of patient problems. Yura and Walsh (1973) describe the nursing assessment as the:

> continuous systematic, critical, orderly, and precise method of collecting, validating, analysing and interpreting information about the physical, psychological and social needs of a patient; the nature of his self-care deficits; and other facts influencing his condition and care.

Gathering information is seen as the initial activity of assessment by Lewis (1968), who adds that a major part of this is in 'the interaction between the nurse and the person, which occurs when there is a meeting of meaning between them'. Organising the collected data assessment forms or frameworks is advocated by most writers: 'A format that is systematic and efficient will be useful for obtaining the greatest amount of information in the shortest time' (Murray, 1976). More importantly, a predetermined framework is said to help in ensuring that all possible patient needs are considered, and none forgotten. Yura and Walsh (1973) use the hierarchy of needs

developed by Maslow as an assessment framework; Abdellah *et al.*
(1960) use a typology of 21 nursing problems they have developed;
Marriner (1979) uses an acronym which acts as a aide-mémoire for
body functions; Pearson and Vaughan (1984a) argue strongly that the
basis for assessment should be a well-developed nursing model; and
Roper *et al.* (1981, 1983), Mayers (1972), Roy (1980) and others all
present assessment formats based on nursing models.

Data are collected, with the close involvement of the patient and
patient problems identified (Tierney, 1984). Campbell (1978) says
that 'for years, nurses have been using medical diseases as the basis
for nursing care. But today, we are developing our own list of patient
problems, which are not diseases, in an effort to establish a more
precise nursing profession'. Some authors use the identified problems
to formulate a 'nursing diagnosis'. Marriner (1975) defines this as 'a
statement or conclusion based on scientific principles and indicating
the patient's need for nursing care'. When problems are identified, a
pattern emerges and the recognition of this pattern leads to a nursing
diagnosis. It establishes both a point of departure and a basis for
nursing care, and the assessment step leads to a 'precise, concise and
highly personalised statement of a nursing diagnosis which will begin
the development of a nursing care plan' (Murray, 1976).

Written, explicit nursing care planning is the next process step.
Stevens (1972) asserts that 'so many credible reasons can be given for
the use of the nursing care plan, that the failure to write plans is
puzzling'. Reasons for written plans include:

1. Nursing must be willing to identify its own content above and
    beyond the carrying out of medical orders.
2. Consensus of nursing approach requires a written plan of care.
3. Continuity, with shift changes, etc., requires a written plan.
4. Patient involvement with his or her own care demands that the
    plan be made explicit.
5. Writing a plan helps the nurse to clarify and solidify her goals.

Setting goals is seen as an integral and important component of care
planning by Marriner (1975), Elhart *et al.* (1978), Mayers (1972) and
Bond (1984).

Implementation is carrying out the plan, and includes
consideration of the method of organising care.

Evaluation is regarded as a crucial, but often forgotten, part of
nursing: 'Whatever the tentative solution or nursing-care plan, the
process is not complete without arriving at some sort of judgement as
to whether the problem has been resolved, unresolved, or created new
problems' (Elhart *et al.* 1978), and evaluation must be continuous and
both formal and informal. Mayers (1972) suggests that evaluation has

been ignored in all health care occupations until recently because 'the mystique associated with all of the healing arts intimidated patients and professionals alike'. She deems it as essential that 'all expected outcomes be evaluated in terms of the goals originally established'.

This systematic, formalised way of delivery care and keeping nursing records was regarded by the group with mixed feelings. They were aware of grave shortcomings in the way care was planned and evaluated at Burford Hospital, with its ignoring of individual patient needs and unacceptable *Nursing Kardex* system. They agreed, in principle, with the idea of using a systematic process; and after two sessions were pleased with their progress in trial assessments and care planning with patients. However, they were worried about the time it took 'writing things down', and needed time to think about a means of introducing such a system. They were adamant that the activities of living, which are listed in the Roper *et al., Model of Nursing* (1980), would be an ideal assessment format, and they were enthusiastic about my suggestion that the group should design an assessment document themselves, using the Roper *et al.* framework if they wished.

Sessions nineteen to twenty-two

The next four sessions followed a different format, and were conducted by a team of professional actors who were experienced in conducting group work using role play. Because they were not health professionals, and identified with patient and lay groups, they aimed at teaching professional practitioners to relate to their clients, from a lay perspective, through empathising with them. The method had been used only once before (I had used it with nurses in another project), and would be an unusual experience for the nurses concerned. The final session was a performance of the theatre company's play, and through that, became known to the national nursing press. As a result of this, the nurses and theatre company had agreed to the presence of a journalist from a nursing journal, and for photographs to be taken at the end. The sessions were therefore looked upon with mixed feelings: the nurses felt apprehensive about the method, but they were excited because it was 'different' and because they thought that the attention being made by the press was 'glamorous' and made them feel important. (The sessions were subsequently reported (Swaffield, 1982) and fulfilled the participants' expectations.)

The method was based on simulating patients by actors. Whitehouse *et al.* (1984) say that patient simulation is a form of role play, in which the role of the patient is taken by a trained simulator, and that of practitioner, by the participants of a training group. 'Role playing involves the spontaneous acting out of roles related to a very distinct group of problems — problems involving human relations' (Schweer, 1972). It involves the group in analysing the behaviours of those playing the roles to increase individual insight into human interaction. Barrows (1971) trained people to act as simulators from various disciplines, Hannay (1980) used trainee social workers, and Meadows and Hewitt (1972) used mothers and professional actors. In all of these reported studies, simulators were 'trained' by the teachers, who were socialised into a professional role. In a sense, these simulators were sophisticated audio-visual aids used by professionals to pass on the ideology of the professional group. The theatre company involved in the sessions for Burford Hospital's nurses had previously developed a different approach which utilised the simulators as lay teachers. Whitehouse *et al.* (1984) describe how the simulator returns to the group after the interaction, and becomes involved in the discussion, at first remaining in the simulated role, and later, out of role. In addition, a member of the company co-leads the group with the professional teacher, to ensure that the lay perspective is emphasised, and the simulators are part of an independent company who develop roles from the basic medical/ nursing/biographical brief given by the professional teacher. Because of this, Whitehouse *et al.* (1984) report that learning centres on attitudes between the professionals and patients, rather than on clinical, 'scientific' aspects. They assert that 'the simulated patients are not just teaching aids structured by medical teachers in a way that consolidates the medical view of patients, but they act as a constant check on untested assumptions about the way patients will act or feel'. The purpose of including this form of learning was to apply the knowledge acquired during the previous sessions of the educational programme; to give the nurses an opportunity actually to see themselves in practice; and to develop a degree of empathy in the participants with the patient culture.

Empathy is defined by La Monica *et al.* (1977) as 'A word which we use when one individual is hearing or understanding another. Empathy involves crawling inside of another person's skin and seeing the world through his eyes. Empathy involves experiencing another person's world as if you were he.' They assert that empathy is the primary ingredient in any helping relationship, a view also expressed by Carkhuff (1969). Murray (1976) and Roper *et al.* (1980) argue for an inclusion of empathy training in basic nurse education.

Rogers (1951) comments on the acquisition of empathic ability. He says that in any helping relationship, the helper must, as far as he/she is able, assume the internal frame of reference of those who are to be helped; perceive the world as they do and communicate this empathic understanding to clients. As the helper communicates warmth and empathy to the client and therefore creates a non-threatening, accepting atmosphere, the relationship can grow and be used in a helpful and constructive way. Alfano (1971) agrees, and reports on the adoption of her concept of 'healing nursing' in a study involving a nursing unit in New York. The concept is based on the development of a close relationship between the nurse and patient, using this closeness to therapeutic effect. The study results show significant improvement in a variety of other settings. Rogers (1951) says that it is difficult to describe how warmth and empathy are communicated and that it is essentially tremendously varied from one person to another. The ability to empathise is therefore, he argues, acquired in a different way by each individual, but has to grow from experience in interacting with others. Direct interaction with real patients, role play between peers and experiences with simulated patients all serve to offer this experience. Yet exposure to actual experience alone is not sufficient. If a student nurse interacts 500 times with a real patient, 500 times with a peer in role play and 500 times with a simulated patient, the ability to empathise is not bound to develop. The essential element of empathy training is said to be feedback (Meadows and Hewitt, 1972; Rutter and McGuire, 1976; Whitehouse *et al.*, 1984).

The participant must have the opportunity to see how he/she interacts with the client; to explore how he/she felt during the interaction; to discover how the patient felt; and to discuss it with a group of interested others. Feedback of this kind has been found to be of crucial importance in the end result of learning taking place. Maguire *et al.* (1978) found that training for medical students in communication was more effective if feedback formed part of the programme. In addition, they found that in those who did receive feedback, either by audio-tape or video, video was significantly more effective and liked.

The Lancet (1981) argued that simulated patients are the most suitable method for such experiential learning exercises. Availability and consistency are seen as their chief advantages, in contrast to patients who are often embarrassed and diffident when being 'used' to train medical staff, and as a consequence, the interaction is atypical and it is difficult to conduct follow-up sessions between the student and patient. Steele and Morton (1978) report that patients 'used' in such a way feel 'like exhibits', their privacy is invaded, and they feel unduly sensitive towards the feeling of the student.

In the method used in the study educational programme, the sessions were based on the use of professional actors identifying with the lay voice, rather than socialised into behaving as a health worker in both role playing and giving feedback. As well, they took a leadership role in the group processes.

Four four-hour sessions were conducted, with seven nurses making up the group, and all having the opportunity to interact with at least two simulated patients each. Twenty-four basic briefs about real patients were given to the theatre company six weeks before the session, to enable the company to assign roles to actors, and for them to develop the roles. The sessions were conducted away from the study hospital, and the mechanics, aims and fine details of the method were explained to the participants a week before the sessions began.

The profiles given to the actors were written in the format given as an example in Figure 6.2.

Frances Johnson is a 23-year-old mother of three, referred from casualty to the clinic for the consultant to see X-rays of hand and spine. She has bruises on the face, painful neck and grossly swollen right hand. Gives a history of having fallen down the stairs. The doctor says that there are no broken bones, and has told her to go into the treatment room to have a crepe bandage applied to her hand.

Frances lives with Andy, her boyfriend, who is not the father of her eldest child. She has lived with him for two years. Recently, he has started to drink heavily, and over the last two months has beaten her a number of times. Last night, he came home at midnight in a violent mood, and punched her repeatedly. This morning he was apologetic and said he was sorry. Frances believes him, but is tired of the violence. She has been unable to tell anyone about Andy's change in behaviour, and makes excuses about her bruises to friends and family. She thinks that Andy's unemployment is the reason for his behaviour − he was sacked from his labourer's job six months ago. She doesn't know what to do and desperately wants to talk to someone she doesn't know, and who is sympathetic.

Fig. 6.2   Patient profile given to actor

Here is how I recorded the performance of this session in my research diary.

Staff Nurse 1 volunteered to do the first interaction − everyone said how brave she was, and there was a good deal of tension, evidenced by giggles, etc.

Frances walked into the treatment room set, and was met by SN1, who was a highly experienced nurse with extensive experience. The actor playing Frances was made up to appear as if she was badly bruised. The nurse carried out the bandaging of the hand, and conversationally elicited a great deal of information. Frances 'hinted' that all was not well, but the nurse proceeded to move away and tidy up. The interaction ended in 6 minutes.

In the follow-up discussion, there was a lot of anxiety. The nurse and the rest of the group said Frances had been beaten up, and wasn't it awful, and what could you do? Frances said she wanted to tell the nurse – she was warm and friendly – but she knew that the nurse didn't want to hear. Lots of discussion – who could she tell, if not the nurse? Is it the nurse's job to pry? What could the nurse do? Is she listening enough? Frances said listening to her would have helped. Out of the role, the actress wanted to know why nurses didn't care as human beings – didn't Frances deserve an ear? Because of the obvious stress in the group (it was the first session), little criticism was made, but it was difficult to end the discussion, because the nurses wanted to talk. 'It happens all the time.' 'It's so real.' 'I didn't know I was like that.'

As the sessions progressed, trust developed and more difficult aspects of nursing relating to patients emerged, and were discussed sensitively, in depth and with increasing openness. By the end session, the group discussions had become long and wide-ranging, and painful personal stories were being shared by the group.

Evaluation of the sessions in a later group meeting evoked entirely positive responses, along with an acknowledgement that they were traumatic and exhausting at the time:

> One of the more reticent nurses had, within a few days, found it possible to over-rule a doctor who had wanted a patient to be kept in the dark about her impending death. She said: 'It was cruel to let her die in the frame of mind she was in – but I couldn't, or at least, wouldn't have pursued the topic with her before the sessions.'

> SN1 said: 'I'm able to talk to relatives now – not happily, but without fear and trembling, having watched my colleagues sort it out in the sessions. And I'm conscious if a patient says he doesn't want something done. I think about why,instead of just persuading him otherwise.
>
> 'I've learned a lot about our own fears. It's something we've all talked about. There are no clear-cut answers, and I always thought there should be. But it's not like that. You can start with your relationship with that patient and work it from there. You're taught for years that there are nurses and patient roles to play, whatever your feelings may be. It's hard to cross that border.
>
> 'Oh, I've learnt so much. About me. About patients. about the others. We're much closer as a team of people, really. And I ache about the way I talk and behave with patients.'

Sessions twenty-two to twenty-four

There were scheduled to take place on the two weeks following the role-playing sessions. However, the group opted to cancel these meetings because they felt a need to come to terms with the learning of the last few weeks. Four weeks after the role plays, two further meetings were held. In the first, the educational programme itself was discussed and evaluated. All comments were positive; all participants expressed a desire to change the work of the hospital, and all participants felt excited about the prospect of such changes. It was agreed that all participants, including me, would commit thoughts for change to writing, and that a further session would be arranged to identify problems which suggested change.

THE DIAGNOSIS – PROBLEMS THAT WARRANTED CHANGES

Although the largest portion of problem identification occurred in the final session, two problems were identified during the six-month educational period, and they were also subject to change planning.

In the second month, the authority discovered that the heating system in the hospital was inadequate, and that they had sufficient funds to install a new boiler. This entailed the evacuation of the hospital building for four months and arrangements were made for in-patients to be transferred to another community hospital 9 miles away, for the casualty department to remain on the hospital site; and for day-patients to be cared for in a vacant building in the mental handicap hospital on the town's outskirts by the existing nursing staff, with additional funds being made available to cover the casualty. This occurrence coincided with frequent discussion in the group of the problems of the ward staff being expected to look after day- and casualty patients, as well as the ward patients, and pre-empted the original strategy to delay any change plans until completion of the educational programme. Within the group, suggested plans were drawn up to modify the building by converting some adjacent outbuildings into a purpose-built day unit, and to upgrade the ward and casualty areas. The plans were accepted as valid by the nursing hierarchy and the Health Authority, but both indicated that they were unwilling, and unable, to provide funds for the building and upgrading, or for any extra staff, who may have been needed if the three areas of work were divided (i.e. wards, casualty, day care). The Hospital's League of Friends, however, were willing to finance the capital costs, and the problem of staffing was discussed in the group. Although they could not see how they could cover the work within their present number, they agreed to report to the nursing hierarchy that an attempt would be made to plan for reorganising the work so that the new buildings could be staffed without extra finance, and that this problem would be one of those identified for inclusion in the change plan which was to be developed by the group. The statement was not initially accepted by the nursing hierarchy, but was eventually, after a meeting between the group and the senior nursing officer. At the end of the first three months of the education programme, the staff were split and dispersed across the three sites, coming together at the group meetings. During the refitting of the heating system, the new day unit was also built, and the casualty area upgraded. Thus the first problem concerning the impinging of other demands on in-patient care was identified, and partial plans were developed and implemented.

The second problem related to the institutional nature of the hospital. Although this was seen as largely attitudinal, the group felt that the physical facilities increased the institutional feeling, and wanted to carpet the ward floors. The League of Friends again agreed to finance this during the closure and to provide a domestic washing machine which would enable the staff to launder personal clothing for patients.

The final group session, devoted to identifying problems which may highlight areas to be changed, lasted 4½ hours and resulted in a list drawn up by all of us. All problems on the list were not unanimously agreed to be valid, but the group decided to accept those which had majority agreement:

1. Patients were currently regarded as recipients of the hospital's expertise and not as part of it.
2. The structure of the staff militated against an alternative way of working.
3. The organisation of care and the patient's day create further oppression of the patient.
4. The role of the nurse, and of nursing itself, was not agreed upon by the nursing staff or understood by other members of the multidisciplinary team.
5. The goals of the nursing team are medically-oriented, and were staff goals rather than patient goals.
6. The current system was unrewarding, monotonous and less beneficial to patients than it could be.

Armed with such a broad list, the group indicated that they were committed to exploring the problems, and constructing a plan for change to be developed from the ideas discussed in the educational programme. The problems were seen as *their* problems, and there was determination to construct a plan which was theirs. The group regarded this as being crucially important. Any changes in the hospital were to be because of a staff-identified/initiated need to pursue thcm and not because of imposition from nurse managers. Furthermore, the group suggested that many of the changes would not meet with the approval of members of the nursing hierarchy, and they suggested that the purpose of the group was to help me persuade others about the plan, and thence bring about the introduction of their own desire changes.

PHASE 2 – ACTION PLANNING

After fifteen months of fieldwork, with nine of these with me as a full-time member of the team, the staff group agreed with much eagerness to plan systematically for making changes in the nursing work in the unit. Action planning entails 'considering alternative courses of action for solving a problem' (Susman and Evered, 1978), and this phase consisted of making specific decisions about actual changes to be made, and testing some of them out. Some were tested by simply asking for responses to suggestions from the staff as a whole, and others by implementing certain plans over a short time, and evaluating their usefulness. The planning phase occurred over a period of nine months.

The process of planning

Restrospective analysis of the subjective data from the daily diary suggested ambivalence among the day nurses when it came to make concrete plans for change. Although the data for phase 1 showed a marked attitudinal change towards the 'new ideologies', following the experiential sessions with the role players, and the group acknowledged the need to change, two members of the group consistently voiced feelings of a sense of loss throughout the planning phase. The prevailing regime was, to them, unsatisfactory, but it was known 'safe' and predictable. The following comments from the day nurses highlight this:

Staff Nurse 1: The place will never be the same again.

Staff Nurse 2: I know – and I really believe – that what you are all saying is right – *really right*. But will it all work, and what happens if it doesn't work? Oh God – it's like being woken up from a deep sleep. I was asleep before and quite happy. Now you've woken us all up, and I can see things wrong that I hadn't noticed before. The question is, which is better? To carry on sleeping and be happy, or to wake up, do things differently and then be happy again. But will I be happy? Still, now that we've got this far, I can't go back to sleep, or at least if I do I'll dream or have nightmares.

Staff Nurse 1: I was looking forward to my retirement and now I couldn't bear to leave because all the changes we are going to make will make it all different, and I'd be so curious about what is going on. I can't leave here until I know it well enough to be able to say to myself: 'Ah, well, they'll be doing so and so now.'

Staff Nurse 2: It will be much better to work with the patients and not for them. But what we've done over the years hasn't been that bad, has it? I mean, I want the new ways, but − well how can I say it? − I sort of like the routine − well, not like it − know it, and will probably long for it in the beginning.

Staff Nurse 1: Of course the doctors shouldn't be so much in control. I've felt that for years. But I'm so used to it, I think I'll miss not being told what to do (if that ever happens, of course!).

Staff Nurse 1: You know, despite Matron's shortcomings, I actually − dare I say it − miss the security of knowing I needn't think or make any decisions. Maybe what I'm saying is, I want to be told what to do, instead of being asked for my opinions (*moans from group, SN3 says: 'six months ago, we all complained about* not *being allowed to think'*) − I *do* want to be involved, and I *do* think that this way is the best. I'm just not used to it and I sometimes find myself wishing I wasn't still working here. I'm not leaving or anything like that, I want to stay − to change, to be part of this whole thing. But − I'm not explaining myself − but better the devil you know ...

These two nurses, however were also very vocal in condemning the old regime, and in urging other group members who occasionally regarded some changes as being too radical, and suggesting slower changes.

Staff Nurse 1: *(to member of group who suggests that only one change at a time should be introduced).* I don't hold with that. We know what needs to be done − we've

	agreed on it − and it's stupid to carry on some of these out-dated, immoral practices, and change only one thing at a time. I say, let's get on with it − I can't wait, really. It's going to be *so* much better.
Staff Nurse 2:	I feel really excited − it's all so challenging. Let's make really good and sensible plans − yes, but let's be enthusiastic and do what we believe in.

Agreeing on specific plans became a predictable, simple process, after a set format for each meeting was arrived at. In the first two meetings, the structure was informal, and few consensus decisions were made. In the second meeting, it was suggested by one nurse that I drew up a list of options, on a range of issues, and that this should form the meetings agenda. The group all agreed that this was the best way to approach the task of planning change, so I drew up the following list of 'choices'.

CHOICES TO BE MADE

1. **A model for practice**
   Choices: Stay the same
   Choose one of those we have learnt about
   Choose a view based on two or more of these learnt about
   Develop one of our own

2. **Using the model**
   Choices   No need to, if we stay the same
   Discuss it with all nurses
   Discuss it with all nurses and ancillaries
   Discuss it with all staff, including doctors, etc.

3. **Using the nursing process**
   Choices: If yes, use documents used in another area
   Base it on a model, and use forms from elsewhere
   Base it on a model, and design our own
   Choices: Involve nurses only in discussion and training
   Also include ancillaries
   Include all of the multidisciplinary clinical team

4. **The patients:**
   (a) *Patient's day* − Stay the same
   Establish new routines
   Have no overall routine, just individual 'routine' for each patient

(b) *Involving patient* − Stay the same
Tell him/her about plan
Nurse and patient do plan together
(c) *Nursing records* − Keep secret (i.e. stay the same)
Show patient
Leave them with patient
(d) *Involving community* − Stay the same
Discuss changes with League of
Friends
Talk to community groups and hold
public meetings

5. **Organising the work**
(a) *Serving departments* − Stay the same
Separate nurse for day care
Separate nurse for day care and
casualty
(b) *Work allocation* − Stay the same
Team nursing
Shift-to-shift allocation of patients to
named persons
Primary nursing
(c) *Accountability* − Nursing officer overall account (i.e. stay
same)
Individual staff nurses to become
accountable

6. **Less specific choices**
(dependent on decisions on above choices)
1. Role of ancillaries
2. Shift hours
3. How best to implement those things we choose

This 'choices' list was used purely as a guideline in group meetings, and was eventually discarded as planning progressed. When it was first introduced, however, none of the group chose to 'stay the same' on any of the issues, and there was fairly rapid agreement on most issues.

CHOICES MADE

Total consensus on an agreed 'new way' was gained. Although no member of the group disagreed on any of the decisions, the two hesitant group members still voiced scepticism on the possibility of the new way ever becoming the new norms.

The Activities of Living nursing model (Roper *et al.,* 1980) was felt to be the most acceptable description of nursing, and was to be explained to all of the 'inside' and 'outside' staff. Nursing process documentation was to be used, and the assessment document based on the activities of living, described in the model was to be designed by the group. All of the nursing notes were to be kept at the patient's bedside, and he/she would have the right to read them at any time. Relatives could read them if the patient gave permission. If he/she was not able to give permission (e.g. due to confusion, unconsciousness, etc.) then relatives could not read them.

The patient's day was to follow his/her usual pattern at home, and no blanket routine imposed. It was impossible, however, to serve lunch and supper at varying times, so these would remain at the established times, but breakfast would be served at any time between 7.30 am and 10.00 am, depending on the patient's preference.

The work was to split up into three main areas: wards, casualty and day care. One of the group opted to become the nurse responsible for day care, and another, to work part-time in casualty. In the evening and at night, ward staff would continue to cover casualty. A system of work organisation based on primary nursing was to be implemented: all direct care was to be given by the nurse; patient autonomy would be promoted; and a generic assistant role would be created by amalgamation of the role of domestic and auxiliary. Finally, a series of public meetings and talks to local groups was planned.

Having reached agreement on these basic issues, a number of discussions to detail what they would actually mean in practice were held, and the overall conclusions recorded in the diary.

THE PATIENTS

The group saw patients as people who, for some reason, were unable to be independent in the activities of living and needed help from nurses in order to become able to return to their own environment. Previously, all patients admitted had been so, ostensibly, for medical reasons, as defined by a doctor. However, all patients admitted since commencement of the study could have easily received more than adequate medical care in their own homes. In the hospital, medical care was no more than that provided by the general practitioners to many others at home. Thus, the sole reason for admission was the need for nursing care. The overall goals of most admissions was a return to home. For those suffering from terminal illness, it was physical, psychological and, to a larger degree, social comfort.

Patients at Burford Hospital needed skilled nursing – with the help of other members of the multidisciplinary team. Routine work and rules had, however, often led to dependence of the patient on the nurses rather than to encouragement of wellness. The majority of patients were able to become much more involved in their care than they currently were.

It was agreed that the patient should be regarded as an autonomous individual with the right to make informed decisions, or to choose to leave such decisions to a health worker. In order for this to be realised in practice, it was planned that:

1. The patient would be asked his/her usual daily living pattern, and that this pattern would be written on a plan of care and followed as nearly as possible.
2. If non-professional carers were involved with the patient at home, they would be at liberty to continue caring within the hospital if they wished (i.e. bathing, feeding, etc.).
3. No secrets would be held by staff, and meaningful teaching was to become a crucial nursing activity, since autonomy in decision-making could only occur if the patient was fully aware of what was happening to him/her. Informed choice cannot be a reality in the uninformed. Nursing notes were to be written in terms intelligible to the layperson and would be on open access by being kept in a special folder at the end of the patient's bed.
4. Patients would be taught how to keep their own charts because handing out drugs from a trolley, filling in secret charts and routinisation all removed opportunities for independence. Patient medicine guides would be supplied to all patients and those capable of doing so would take their own medications.
5. Visiting hours were to be abolished and 24-hour visiting would be established.
6. Patient autonomy could only be realised if the nurse, who was present 24 hours a day, had the power to allow patients to make their own decisions. The role of the nurse as key worker and the legitimate on-the-spot decision-maker was to be negotiated.
7. All blanket routines, other than cooked meal-times, were to cease.

NURSING

As patients were primarily admitted for nursing, the activities of nursing were central to the goals of Burford Hospital. Nursing was seen as a complex activity based on the development of a close, helping relationship between nurse and patient, and focused on the patient's subjective experiences concerning his/her current state, and on enabling independence on the activities of living.

For the nursing to operate in this way, it was planned to pursue the following:

1. Have three full-time nurses in post by reducing the hours of one of the nurses. The latter would take over the running of the casualty between 9.00 am and 4.00 pm.
2. Change the shift system so that the full-time nurses worked only 8.00 am – 4.30 pm and part-time nurses either 5.00 – 9.00 pm or 9.00 pm – 8.00 am.
3. The full-time nurses would be designated as primary nurses, carrying a defined caseload of patients.
4. The part-time nurses would be designated as associate nurses.
5. On any given day, one full-time nurse would be on a day off, leaving two nurses to care for nine patients.
6. All patients would be *referred* to the nurses, and not admitted by a doctor. On referral, a nursing assessment of the patient would determine whether or not he/she could be helped by the hospital; whether the current workload was such that admission was feasible, and thus, whether or not to admit.
7. Decision to discharge would ultimately be jointly made by the patient, his family and the nurses.
8. Physiotherapists and social workers were to be used as a consultant to nurses. Such workers would teach patient and nurse the course to be pursued and this would be carried out by the nurse, except when it was outside her competence, or not feasible because of time (e.g. all walking exercises, etc. were to be carried out by nurses, but the physiotherapist would continue to administer ultrasound treatment).

THE NURSES

Job descriptions for the new nursing roles were prepared, and the following provides a summary of the duties.

The primary nurse

Each primary nurse worked full-time, and the duty roster was structured so that two primary nurses would always be on duty. Each would be allocated patients on admission, and be totally responsible for their nursing care until discharge, as well as ensuring home care is provided where relevant. Each would therefore have three patients to look after, and act as an associate nurse to her off-duty colleague by caring for her patients. Total responsibility included: assessing the needs of the patient; compiling a written care plan with the patient; giving all care while on duty; and evaluating the effects of the plan. When off-duty, the carrying out and evaluation of the written care plan would be delegated to the associate nurse, but alteration of the care plan remained the responsibility of the primary nurse. Each primary nurse was to be provided with a long-range radio-pager so that she could be contacted. Accountability for nursing throughout the hospital stay was to be vested in the primary nurse, and she would communicate with the patient's family and those members of the multidisciplinary clinical team involved.

The associate nurse

Because the development of a close nurse–patient relationship was seen as fundamental to effective care planning, the limited contact possible when working 20 or less hours a week was said to be insufficient to enable part-time nurses to act as primary nurses. All part-time nurses were designated as associate nurses. The associate nurse was to be accountable for carrying out care prescribed in the written care plan and to feed back evaluation to the primary nurse through writing progress notes; giving verbal reports and contacting the primary nurse directly using the radio-pager in urgent situations.

Communication between nurses

The 'hand-over report session', held at each shift change in the ward office, was to be abandoned. At each shift change, the nurse going off duty was to report to the nurse taking over care of the individual patient, at the patient's bedside, so that he/she was included in the information exchange.

The nursing officer

The role of the nursing officer was seen as expert consultant in nursing practice, who could be consulted on clinical matters, and who would arrange the environment to allow primary and associate nurses to function. As in all process of consultation, his advice could legitimately be accepted or rejected by the primary nurse, who in the final analysis was accountable for the patient's care.

THE NON-NURSING MEMBERS OF THE MULTIDISCIPLINARY CLINICAL TEAM

The doctor

The doctor was seen as an expert in diagnosing and treating disease, and as an equal colleague to the nurse. He would be expected to relate to the appropriate primary nurse for each of the patients he was attached to, and to make decisions about medical treatment.

The domestic assistant and nursing auxiliary

These two categories of worker were to be regraded as a single, generic assistant, known as a 'care assistant'. This role was to encompass keeping the environment clean, and to *assist* the nurse in giving care, both by getting equipment ready and giving physical assistance when two people were needed. The care assistant role was not to include giving care in place of a nurse (e.g. they would not be asked to bath or dress a patient, but may help the nurse to do this, or run the bath).

The social worker

The role of the social worker was one of advising the nurse by producing social reports on request, and to take over from the care when patients had social problems beyond her competence.

The physiotherapist

The physiotherapist was to work in a similar way to the social worker.

The district nurses and health visitor

These nurses were to be based in the hospital, and to act as consultant to the hospital nurses on admission, and on discharge planning.

THE ACTION PLAN

The action plan fell into two distinct areas. For some of the changes, the group wished to introduce them immediately and assess their usefulness or feasibility before deciding on how to incorporate them into a long term strategy. Other changes were seen as fundamental to the overall change in direction of the unit.

Changes in the patient's day fell into this 'try out immediately' category, and it was decided to explain and discuss the rationale behind this to all of the staff, and try to begin it on a limited basis to assess what was and what was not possible before drawing up specific targets. It was agreed that patients would only be woken up at the times they requested, and go to bed when they wished. The routine afternoon rest period would also be discontinued, and the 'deadline' for completion of bedmaking abandoned.

These ideas were discussed at a meeting with the night and evening nurses, and at one arranged with the domestics and auxiliaries. The suggestions were met with some hostility by the night nurses.

The night nurses (who had already participated in a three-day workshop on the underlying principles of the proposed changes) indicated that they were threatened by the proposed changes. Allowing patients to sleep beyond 6.30 am would lead, they said, to a feeling of guilt:

NN1   What happens if they all want to sleep till 8 am? The day staff would think we'd done nothing.

NN2:   The day staff may say that's OK, but there'll be many a sly dig if they walk on and everybody's still asleep.

NN1:   How will we get the night work done then?

Researcher: What night work do you mean?

NN1:   Well, the medicines, the washes and things?

Researcher: Well, it wouldn't be night work anymore – it would be continuous work, to be done by whoever is there when the patient needs help.

NN1:   Ha! And what do the day staff think of that then?

The evening nurses, present at the same meeting, were less concerned about allowing patients to stay up in the day room than the night nurses were about allowing patients to stay in bed. The night nurses, however, were also unhappy about having to help patients to bed when they came on duty. The needs of patients were not considered in any of the discussion by night nurses. They were, however, very concerned about 'helping the day staff' and about the morality of each shift fulfilling its obligations to 'getting the work done'.

A second meeting was organised, to bring together the night nurses and the day nurses. This second meeting began with a presentation of the data collected in phase 1, which was about the work of the night nurse. These data suggested that the night nurses had a minimal workload for coming on duty at 9.00 pm, until about 6.00 am the following morning, when they were required to complete an enormous amount of tasks before the day staff arrived at 8.00 am. They had to:

- Wake every patient.
- Take everyone's temperature.

- Give everyone a cup of tea.
- Give everyone a wash.
- Change wet or dirty beds.
- Give medications (including injections).
- Serve breakfasts.
- Tidy ward and all service rooms.

It was suggested that this approach was similar to the evening shift, when all patients had to be helped to bed. Furthermore, the night nurses had to dispense night sedations and milk drinks at 9.00 pm with the lights out and patients already settled.

The day staff suggested that the changes did not create any more or less work for the night nurse — it simply moved it around. Instead of little work at night, and lots in the morning, it led to more work at night, and little in the morning. After much discussion, the night nurses accepted that they would try to work this way for a limited period, but repeated their concern that the day staff 'won't be suited when they come on and see us sitting down waiting for patients to wake up'.

The discussion on these feelings lasted 1½ hours!

DN1: Why feel guilty when we've all agreed that we should work like this.

NN1: Because you know why. If we've been busy and haven't got all the breakfasts out when the day staff come on, what happens?

DN1: I dunno, what?

NN1: You soon let us know.

DN1: Do we?

NN1: Yes, it's not what you say to us — it's things like: 'Oh, breakfasts not out yet?' Or: 'It's suddenly got busy then, hasn't it?'

NN2: Yes, I said that the other morning, but there was only six patients, and I couldn't see why you'd been so busy.

NN1: Well, we'd had two casualties, that's why.

Researcher: Maybe we don't really feel that we can trust each other enough to believe that we'll all work as hard as we could if there aren't set jobs to be done.

DN1: That's just it. We're more interested in making sure we all pull our weight than in doing what patients need. What's this hospital here for? To suit the staff, or to suit the patients?

NN1 To suit the staff at the moment, but it should be to suit the patients.

DN3: I think we could get it so that it suits both.

Rivalry between shifts about completing work was argued about, laughed at and finally acknowledged to be unnecessary, and it was resolved to introduce the change the next week.

Two weeks later, at another meeting between day, evening and night nurses, progress was discussed and evaluated. The night staff still felt some discomfort about not waking patients, especially on two mornings when all of the patients slept through until the day staff arrived:

NN: I felt a real fraud (*laughter*). I had to sit on my hands when it got to 7.00 am and I told Marie (*auxiliary*) to go and make a noise in the kitchen to disturb somebody. But I think it's much better. Fred sleeps ever so well now that he goes to bed later, and we've more chance of getting to know the patients when they're all awake when we come on. But I shall *never* get used to not running around in the morning.

One of the day nurses, however, was uncomfortable about having to serve breakfasts, and said it 'slowed up' the work:

SN1: It has put all the work back, and really slowed us up. We didn't get the beds finished until 12 one day last week.

SN2: But we said it doesn't matter when the beds are finished — you know, 'getting the work done' mentality is something we're trying to shift.

SN1: I *know*. But I hate it — I can't stand having stripped, unmade beds in the ward. It makes me feel disorganised.

It was agreed, however, that the approach was better for patients, and to continue with it.

The auxiliaries and domestics were quite happy with the suggested change when it was discussed at the first meeting, but they were critical at a meeting two weeks after the change was introduced. Their unhappiness was with the loss of a clear routine, which they saw as a drop in standards, and a sign of 'things slipping':

'You've got to have discipline and routine, or put up with shoddy work.'

'I like to know exactly what had to be done, and I'll do it. If you leave it to patients, they'll keep changing their minds, and you won't know whether you're coming or going.'

'It's getting too lax for me, and it won't be long before you see things slipping.'

Although they agreed to carry on with the flexibility, they made it clear that they did not agree with it.

The other changes desired by the staff group were incorporated into a systematic plan of action, which comprised informing everyone about the changes and securing the needed resources. It was felt that introducing an aspect of change each week or gradually, would lead to confusion, and that a clean break between the 'old' and the 'new' would be more conducive to proclaiming the 'new ideology'.

The proposed plan (Figure 6.3) was discussed at length with all of the nursing staff, and the domestics and nursing auxiliaries.

July 1982: Meetings to discuss changes with:
- all nurses
- all domestic and auxiliaries
- nurse management
- cook and porter
- physiotherapist
- social worker
- doctors
- administrator
    Order needed materials, i.e. uniforms
                                    nursing notes
                                    note holders
                                    medicine charts and
                                    cabinet
                                    additional stationery
    Negotiate with individuals about new off-duty arrangements, and changes in job descriptions and contracts where necessary.

Move back to main site (mid-July)

August 1982:   Iron out any difficulties or queries, and modify plans in response to meetings.

Bank Holiday Monday: All nursing staff on duty, and commence adoption of new roles, uniform shifts, work patterns and documentation.

September 1982 onwards:
    Set up weekly meetings to discuss progress, evaluate changes, and modify according to experience. Make further plans for change.

August 1983: Evaluate nursing work in the unit formally.

Figure 6.3   Agreed change plan

Final agreement on the plan was met with euphoria by all of the group who had been involved throughout the project todate:

SN1: Now that we know what we are doing, I am pretty sure that we'll manage it.

SN2: Isn't it exciting?

SN3: I feel like a member of a revolutionary party who's just about to pull off the revolution.

SN4: I can't wait for 'D-day'. (*referring to 31 August*)

Most of them suggested that the future was challenging and exciting, and made little reference to any possible difficulties, although the nurse who began working at the hospital after the study commenced repeatedly urged the group to recognise that it wouldn't be easy at the beginning, and believing that it would be easy would make it 'depressing' when difficulties arose:

'I'm excited and enthusiastic as well, but I bet it isn't as easy as it sounds.'

'I think we should be prepared for some people to play up when we change, you know. If we expect it, then we will be more likely to be able to cope with problems.'

'I'm telling you now, the doctors won't like it and once we start, they'll start getting at us. So I think we should be ready for it, and not get upset or revert back as soon as one of them says it doesn't work. (*To group member who says that everybody has said they are really excited about the change*) Yeah, but the doctors haven't, and it's one thing for the others to say with their mouths that they like the ideas, but another thing when it affects the way they behave at work.'

The general feeling in the group was of optimism and anticipation. The part-time nurses and night staff also indicated that they were enthusiastic, and were apparently pleased that the plan had been developed by 'them'. Despite their non-attendance at most of the group meetings, they felt that the three-day workshop and the meetings to discuss their reactions to the plan involved them enough to enable them to identify themselves as co-producers of the plan.

The information meetings I was to organise were to be attended by as many of the group of six nurses who had been continuously involved as possible.

7 | Changing Burford

PHASE 3: ACTION-TAKING

Because of the installation of the new boilers, the action planning phase was happening when the hospital was working on three separate sites. As well as the planned changes derived from the action research process, a number of other changes, such as the physical facilities in the hospital building being upgraded and reorganised, were also occurring because of forces from outside the group. A new, purpose-built day hospital had been created from some disused outbuildings, the minor casualty area had been transformed from two sparsely furnished rooms into a purpose-designed treatment area and minor theatre; the bed complement had been increased from 9 to 12; and the ward areas had been carpeted and decorated. (The three additional beds were not, however, to be opened until phase 5.)

Because of the reorganisation of floor-space, the staff room, which had previously been adjacent to the ward, had been moved to a room upstairs, and a reception area in the hallway had been created. All of these apparently minor changes were seen by the staff to offer both a new start and some need to organise the work to accommodate the different layout of patient and staff areas. The situation seemed ideal for the first steps in action-taking, which was to inform all of the inside staff and outside staff about the action plan, and to discuss its implementation. Everyone knew that the hospital was different physically and wanted to talk about what this would mean in terms of changing certain aspects of the work:

Doctor: We need to get together soon, before the move back, to discuss these extra beds, and to get the new day hospital and casualty off to a good start.

Domestic: Hoovering carpet instead of polishing the floor is going to be harder work — so we all want a meeting to negotiate how we'll manage.

There was a general feeling that the new, transformed hospital deserved a new, transformed look and a general desire to explore how to get the best out of it. The proposed meetings were therefore well accepted, with some individual requests for a meeting being made before staff were asked. Some staff had also resigned, thus creating vacancies to be filled. One part-time staff nurse left because she disliked the relaxation in rules ('I can't work in a place with such low discipline') and a nursing auxiliary resigned for similar reasons.

The meetings with the various staff groups included in the action plan were a natural prelude to the move back by the staff, and were well accepted.

NURSES

The six nurses on day duty had been fully involved in the previous phases, while the night nurses and evening nurse had only been involved in a comparatively short series of workshops, but had participated in preparing the action plan. The meeting arranged with the nurses were therefore merely reviewing the plan and agreeing that it was still acceptable. Details were discussed and agreed upon. Primary nurses were to wear a uniform with a different coloured trim from associate nurses, and it was agreed after much discussion that the current uniform policy should be relaxed. This policy required nurses to wear brown or black lace-up shoes, brown or black tights/stockings, and no jewellery other than a wedding ring and gold studs if a nurse's ears were pierced. The nurses felt that it was important to avoid a uniformity, even though a uniform dress was worn:

'Uniformity strips us of our individuality and makes us sort of non-persons.'

'We need to appear a bit more informal if the place is to be more homely, really.'

The suggestion that uniforms be abandoned, however, was only regarded positively by one nurse:

'Oh, no, nobody would know we were nurses!'

'The patients feel more secure with nurses in uniform.'

'They expect to see nurses in uniform.'

'I need to wear something which I can take off and wash after work – our own clothes would be ruined.'

'Wearing uniform is a great leveller. If I had to choose something to wear every day, I'd be thinking: "Oh no – I wore that yesterday" – but wearing a uniform means you don't have to think.'

The one dissenter argued that nurses should take thought about their appearance and what they wore: 'After all, we would if we were going to meet people in a pub, or have visitors at home – how come the patients don't deserve that?' The group agreed to compromise with everyone wearing a uniform dress, but with the freedom to wear shoes and stockings/tights of their own choice.

Sample of note folders, which could be hung at the end of the patient's bed, but designed so that notes were not on open view, were discussed and one design was selected, as were the new charts and medicine cabinet.

The two full-time nurses were selected as primary nurses, and the part-time nurse agreed to a full-time position as the third primary nurse. The planned off-duty changes were agreed upon, and the new job descriptions accepted.

An evening nurse had her reservations about the primary and associate roles, and the rest of the group understood her feelings and attempted to handle them:

EN: I can't see why you need a trained nurse on in the evenings if all there is to do is to carry out precise instructions written by the primary nurse in the care plan. I feel as if I'm just going to be a dog's body.

SN1: But you won't be. You'll be responsible for carrying out the plan, yes, but you will be using your expertise to do that.

EN: I know, but it's sort of insulting. A trained nurse should *know* what the patient needs, and not have to have it written down.

SN1: Give us an example of what you mean.

EN: Well, if Mr Bloggs is bedfast and incontinent, any trained nurse should know to turn him two-hourly and treat his pressure areas.

SN2: Of course you would know that – but you might not know, for instance, that his left leg hurts when he's turned, and you should be supported; or that he's been using Vaseline on his bottom for twenty years and he thinks it works.

EN: Well, I could ask him, you know.

SN1: Yes, but then it ends up with him being asked the same thing at every shift change, or, more often than not, him not being asked, and having a different potion slapped on him each time.

EN: Well, I'm not going to argue about it, but I'm not sure how happy I'll be. Whenever I've been on in the evening, I've been

in charge, and used my judgement on what is best for the
patient.

SN2: And you've done that really well. It's just that, well, what we
are really trying to do is to let the patient be in charge, if he is
able.

EN: No you're not − you're making the primary nurse in charge,
even when she's not there.

SN1: Yes, it does look like that, doesn't it? But it isn't really. You
see, the primary nurse is there for 8 hours a day, 5 days a week
with the patient; and she is there when most things happen.
Like, when the doctor comes, when physio is organised, and
things. Because of this, she gets quite close to the patient, and
negotiates things with him, you see. In real life, the patient
won't really get his say without him being able to relate to his
own nurse. It's not an ego trip for the primary nurse − it's a
try at upping the patient.

EN: And how do you know this then, considering we haven't tried
it yet?

SN1: Well, we don't. But that's why we want to try it. It sort of
sounds right, but it might flop completely.

EN: Well, I hope it does.

This particular nurse (who, incidentally, resigned nine months later)
voiced her disapproval throughout the meeting, and felt that the part-
time nurses were being discriminated against by not being allowed to
be primary nurses. The group as a whole, however, felt strongly that
nurses working 20 hours or less a week, usually in four-hour shifts,
would not be able to develop sufficient relationships with patients to
enable them to fulfil the primary nurse role. The other part-time
evening and night nurses felt that at that time they were either unable
or unwilling to invest more of their time or energy to nursing itself,
and that they would be happy with the responsibility of implementing
and evaluating care planned by someone else, and in making on-the-
spot decisions within the parameters of the plan.

The previously high optimism was, however slightly lower, and the
group indicated that they were beginning to feel a mixture of
excitement, and uncertainty.

'The sooner we get it started, the better.'

I don't know how I feel now. Part of me is excited, part of me is sceptical
and part of me is too lazy to handle all this.'

'I want it to be done; then I'll let you know my feelings.'

The overall climate of the meetings with the nurses was, although
mixed, positive and expectant. Change was wanted, but the energy to

bring it about was a worry to some, and a degree of cynicism lay under
the apparent enthusiasm. One day nurse, who was to become a full-
time primary, appeared to want to support the changes in group
discussion, but was much less approving in one-to-one conversation:

> 'It all sounds good, doesn't it, but it might be a lot of fuss about nothing.
> A way to make things a bit more exciting in a pretty boring job.'

> 'Primary nursing, partnership, nursing process, and "the right of the
> individual" are all OK. But we're talking about incontinent, smelly
> geriatrics, and tarting it all up won't change that.'

> 'Find me a rich man, and I'll be off tomorrow. I work because of the
> money – no more. And you can't tell me that anybody else doesn't. These
> new ideas are all very well, but I'll have to do more – and there'll still be
> no more money.'

> 'I believe in it all, for me – I mean, if I was the patient, I'd like it. But I
> want an easy life as a nurse, so you'll have a hard job changing me!'

When these sort of remarks were raised in the group, they were denied
by the 'doubting' nurse, and quickly criticised and discarded by the
rest of the group.

ANCILLARY STAFF

Because the nursing auxiliaries regarded themselves as nurses, and
not, at this stage, of similar status to the domestics, meetings were
held separately for the two groups.

Nursing auxiliaries

The total action plan was met with some criticism by this group. They
were prepared to be renamed as 'care assistant' as long as their salary
and conditions of service remained as nursing auxiliaries. The
suggestion that all direct care be given by the nurses was not
welcomed.

> 'What will we do, if the nurses do that?'

> 'Oh, come on, it doesn't need a trained nurse to give a bedpan.'

> 'I came into this job to be a nurse – and that's what I intend to be.'

> 'It sounds as if we are going to be made redundant.'

The auxiliaries felt competent in giving nursing care, and saw their
role as being superior to the domestic, with one describing how hard

she had worked to gain 'promotion from a cleaner to an auxiliary nurse'. Two of the group had commenced nurse training, with one discontinuing after 8 months, and another after 16 months, and both argued that they were well qualified to give total patient care. The atmosphere of this first meeting with this group was one of resistance to any change, a strong desire to maintain the status quo, and a loud argument that the nursing auxiliary should be the 'real' nurse, and qualified nurses should carry out medically-oriented tasks and direct the auxiliaries. The auxiliaries were only four in number, and worked only on night duty, and had only been in post for two years. Prior to that, night duty was covered by one registered nurse working alone, who could call the matron who lived in the flat on the first floor of the hospital. There was a general view among the staff, therefore, that having two people on duty at night was really quite wasteful − the workload was light, and the nursing auxiliary was largely there because of safety. Furthermore, the domestics on day duty were in reality carrying out more nursing duties than the nursing auxiliaries. They wore the same uniform too, but were paid considerably less, had poorer conditions of service and described themselves as domestics to the local community. It was quite understandable that the auxiliaries felt threatened by this state of affairs, and wanted the domestics on day duty to do domestic work only, and the hospital to employ day duty nursing auxiliaries to give care. The action plan conflicted directly with their aspirations associated with gaining recognition that the auxiliary was the true bedside nurse, with greater status than the untrained domestic.

The group also laid great store on the need for a clear hierarchy and emphasised the need for 'respect to seniors':

'I don't hold with Christian names. If I called the staff nurse Mary, I'd lose respect for her.'

'I respect my seniors, and the domestics should do the same.'

'When I was younger, you stood up if the sister or staff nurse came into the room. There's nothing wrong with that kind of respect. If you know your place, the work gets done more efficiently.'

In line with this, all agreed that if they were *told* that they *had* to act as assistants to nurses, then 'we'll jolly well have to do it'.

Domestics

In direct contrast to the nursing auxiliaries, the domestics were strongly in favour of the proposals. They saw them as giving recognition to the fact that, as a group, the domestics did assist nurses, and that they were no different from the nursing auxiliaries:

Dom 1:   We do more nursing than the auxiliaries, but we've had no
         training, and the nurses would be better at it than us.
Dom 2:   Well, the auxiliaries haven't had any training either.
Dom 3:   Some of them have.
Dom 2:   Yeah, but they didn't finish the training – and you don't
         have to have any training to be an auxiliary. We're
         untrained; they're untrained. We are no different really.
Dom 1:   Don't get me wrong. I would be miserable only doing the
         cleaning. I think we should be like care assistants. Keep the
         place clean and give the nurses a hand. But not doing the
         nursing. It's not fair on the patient, and not on us.

Both groups were given a draft care assistant's job description and a
care assistant's manual, and both were enthusiastic about a
suggestion that a series of in-service lectures on items in the manuals
should be conducted.

Doctors

Three meetings were held with the three doctors from the associated
practice, the proposed primary nurses and myself. The senior partner
had worked in the hospital for over thirty years, while the two other
partners had joined within the last four years. All agreed that change
was needed in the hospital. Both the junior partners agreed with all of
the proposed changes, but the senior partner disagreed with some of
them. The senior partner, in particular, felt strongly that he was in
charge of 'his' patients, and the role of the nurse was to support him
in the medical regime. The way this doctor cared for patients was
different from the others in that he was less interested in scientific
medicine, and was holistic in his approach to care (although, when
this was suggested to him, he dismissed the term as jargonistic and
asserted that he was a 'scientific doctor'!). Nevertheless, he knew the
patients and their families well, took the elderly out on car rides at the
weekend, and was known by the community as a 'caring doctor'. His
objections to the action plan related to the access of records to
patients:

'They are my records, and aren't the patients' business.'

'If I knew they would see them, then I wouldn't write what I thought.'

'They wouldn't understand them, so what is the point?'

He also felt strongly that I, as the nursing officer, should control
work because the registered nurses were not 'able to take

responsibility'. He approved, however, the changes proposed in the patient's day; community involvement; home visits by the nursing officer prior to admission; greater involvement of the nursing officer in policy-making and clinical decision-making; more systematic nursing assessment; and the reorganisation of work. Blunt in his contributions to the discussions, he was honest and frank in his opinions. Since the beginning of the study, the senior partner had increasingly relied on nursing opinion, and often expressed his satisfaction in having a male nursing leader.

The other two partners loudly supported the action plan in its entirety, and the senior partner bowed to their opinions, and the plan was accepted. The three meetings considered how the plan was to be implemented, and focused on open records. The proposal initially referred only to nursing notes, but the two younger doctors expressed the wish to include their records in the open system. Because of the senior partner's reluctance to the idea, the mechanics of this had to be discussed at length. At this stage in the action plan, the doctors were not only supportive, but also, in some ways, enthusiastic. The data from the diary suggest, however, that much of this positiveness related to their perception of my own capabilities, rather than nursing itself.

The doctors regarded the other nurses as requiring constant supervision, because nurses 'always need to be led', and as subject to emotion and irrational behaviour, because 'nurses are women'. I was regarded differently, and related to in a different way. Although this may have been associated in part with my academic links, the fact that I was male seemed to be more significant:

'I did have my doubts about a male matron, but the logic of a male mind is really showing.'

'If you can get them to think like you, it'll work well.'

'It's just like our surgery staff − they'll always fight among each other, when you have a lot of women working together. You've got to have leadership to hold them together.'

They viewed the proposed changes as a worthwhile exercise of the application of male logic to a situation previously led by women. The senior partner warned the third meeting, however, that:

'A lot of this is lefty stuff, you know. If you got rid of that, it would be OK.'

Other personnel

The other staff who were not part of an occupational group were talked with individually. The physiotherapist agreed with all of the action plan, as did the cook, social worker and occupational therapist.

INTRODUCING THE FIRST MAJOR CHANGES

As the information meetings were well received and the change plans agreed to, all of the necessary equipment was obtained, and off-duties were planned to enable the staff to introduce the main changes on one designated day. This came to be known as 'D-Day', and was joked about and a frequent topic of conversation in the weeks before. The staff would return to the upgraded unit three weeks before 'D-day'. On the day itself, the new uniforms and shifts were adopted; the patients' day was modified; and all patients contributed to an assessment and a formulation of their own care plan, and to taking their own medication. In the first three weeks, I gave support and then gradually withdrew it. Four weeks after the change, the diary observation were collated to provide a description of the hospital's work, before commencing the weekly review meetings.

THE 'NEW' WORK NORMS

After four weeks, the typical working day was observed to be as follows:

8 am: Two day nurses on duty: each day nurse takes brief handover report about patient she is to care for *only*, from the night nurse. If the patient is awake, this took place with the patient.

NN: Mrs A, your nurse has just come on, and we need to tell her about how you've got on through the night.
Mrs A: Oh, hello Sue!
NN: Well, I've written that you fell asleep about 11 o'clock, after that cup of tea, and that you called me at 6 for painkillers. Your pain was 5 on the painometer, and you said you've had a good night.
Mrs A: Yes, that's about it.
DN: Well, that's an improvement, isn't it? I'll come back in a minute after I've had the rest of the report, to sort out today's programme.

As patients woke, breakfast was given to each. After the report, each day nurse discussed plans for the day with each of her assigned patients, and then the nurses and care assistants had a cup of tea in the kitchen while patients ate breakfast. At this time, a care assistant was assigned to work with each nurse, and the morning's plans were discussed. Following this, no steady routine was adhered to.

Although most patients did get up and dressed, some did not, and some slept until 10–11 am. All work with patients was carried out by the nurse, and the care assistants helped when requested, but spent most of the time making empty beds, fetching things for the nurse, and cleaning. Patients were bathed either in the morning or afternoon, depending on their preference. A doctor attended each weekday morning and saw each of the nurses, and went with them to see patients when necessary.

12 mid-day: Patients were asked whether they wished to eat at the table or by their own beds, and the meal was served by the patient's own nurse. Medications were given by the nurse when the patient was unable to do so independently. Otherwise, the patient was given his/her own lockable drawer at medicine time, and took the appropriate medication while the nurse watched. At 12.30 pm, one nurse went for lunch, and at 1.30 pm the other. The care assistants finished duty at 2.30 pm, leaving two nurses on the ward.

Afternoon: A number of various activities were carried out, but again, these were unpredictable and dependent upon patients' preferences. On the whole, the afternoon was a time for talk between nurses and patients, and the writing of nursing records. Patients who wished to read their own notes tended to do so during this period.

4.15 pm: One evening nurse and one care assistant on duty. Report given by patient's nurse, with patient involved. Day nurses off at 4.30 pm.

Evening: The only fixed activity was the serving of supper, carried out with the help of volunteers from the community. Some patients were then bathed, some helped to bed, others stayed up.

8.45 pm: Night nurse on duty – report at bedside again. Milk drinks served and medications given or supervised. Patients put to bed, etc. according to preferences.

Morning: Patients were not woken by the night staff. Those who did wake were given breakfast and medications, and others left to sleep. Because the mornings were dark, few patients woke before the day staff came on duty, and the night nurses tended to sit in the duty room, waiting for patients to stir.

On referral from the doctor, district general hospital, district nurse, etc., the patient's information was recorded on a referral form (Appendix X). Then, if the need was urgent, a decision made to accept or reject was made then and there, and otherwise a visit to the patient was arranged. The latter option involved a visit to the patient's home, and assessment of nursing needs using a home assessment form (Appendix XI). Following assessment a further decision was made. In this way, all admissions were judged by a nurse in order to determine whether or not the major needs were for nursing, and whether or not the unit could effectively meet these needs. In the first four weeks, eleven referrals were made. Of these, eight were accepted; two were rejected and the doctor was advised to refer to the acute hospital because the unit was unable to meet those patients' individual needs; and one was referred to social services, who arranged admission to a bed in a 'landlady scheme' on the same day.

Patients admitted were assigned a primary nurse. On admission, this nurse would begin to collect information about the patient in order to assess needs, and would draw up a written plan of care. This was kept in a folder, with medical and other notes, at the patient's bedside, and the patient was encouraged to contribute to the care plan. The fairly comprehensive records were not referred to at this point by the doctors, but were used extensively by the paramedical staff. Associate nurses followed the care plans, but, if this was not possible, reasons were stated in the progress notes. These progress notes were also used to write in evaluative comments about the care planned, and its outcome.

Within four weeks the new system of working was virtually institutionalised and seen as the norm. The staff said they liked it, patients were positive and the paramedical workers had no criticisms. On the first group meeting, however, the following conflict areas were identified:

1. The primary nurses were finding it difficult to nurse terminally ill patients in a close partnership way because the doctors sometimes chose not to inform patients of their diagnosis, and insisted that the nurses should do the same.
2. The primary nurses found it difficult to act as key workers when doctors passed on information to patients without including the nurse.
3. The doctors did not like the build-up of paperwork in the case folders.
4. The doctors did not like having to find the right nurse, and wanted a return to having one nurse taking them round the patients.
5. The nurses as a whole felt that the doctors were devaluing their role, and still saw themselves as leader of a multidisciplinary team.

Following this meeting, it was decided to conduct a series of workshops for the multidisciplinary team using the theatre group used in phase 1. As the practical implementation of the new norms appeared to be satisfactory, it was felt that the major problems presented at the meeting arose from difficulties in relationships between staff, and role-perception gaps between nurses and doctors.

The new norms were maintained, and the workshop series organised to take place sixteen weeks after the introduction of the changes.

INTERDISCIPLINARY LEARNING

A total of eleven sessions were organised, over a period of six weeks, and three doctors, four primary nurses, one district nurse and one health visitor from the unit were asked to participate. A further doctor, three district nurses and three health visitors from outside the unit were invited to attend, so that the group of sixteen participants consisted of:

- Four primary nurses
- Four district nurses
- Four health visitors
- Four doctors

The information letters sent to the participants are given in Appendix XIII. The plan was to conduct patient-centred sessions, using simulated patients and group discussion, as in phase 1. The participants were from different areas, so that the focus was on how the team as a whole affects the patient and on the roles of doctors and nurses.

The first four sessions were 'single-discipline': one session was for the four primary nurses, one for the general practitioners, one for the health visitors and one for the district nurses. It was felt that this would introduce the method those participants who had no previous exposure, which was everyone but the primary nurses, as well as allowing each group to look at their own specific role.

The next four sessions were for four, small, mixed groups, each with a doctor, primary nurse, district nurse and health visitor.

The third series was for two large mixed groups, with two from each discipline.

The final session was for discussion, evaluation and specifying learning.

Attendance was good, with only one participant dropping out (a local GP who was unwilling to give his reasons) after the small mixed group. Although each session revolved around a patient, all of the difficulties brought up in the meeting were discussed, and the philosophy of the unit was repeatedly brought up, heatedly debated and increasingly understood.

The final session, was for all participants, and 14 out of 15 attended. All were asked to complete an open-ended questionnaire (Appendix XIV) and this was used as the framework for the discussion.

This session was marked by the eagerness of the participants to discuss the impact of the sessions on their own attitudes, and how this should influence future team work in the unit. Most participants felt anxious prior to all sessions, because they feared 'showing myself up'. They all, however, felt they had learnt something, while two health visitors who were not from the unit felt that the sessions had been traumatic and they would not be prepared to participate in similar experiences again. The mixed groups were said to be the most beneficial, and all of the non-primary nurses expressed the view that they did not realise how hospital nurses in the Burford unit worked *with* patients until they participated in the sessions. The doctors loudly expressed the view that, through the sessions, they had come to realise how central the primary nurse's role was to patient care in the unit.

After much light-hearted discussion, the group as a whole presented a number of axioms to guide future working relationships within the unit:

1. The primary nurse should be seen as the 'key worker' and her notes as the most crucial and patient-centred. (Moreover, the doctors suggested that medical notes be abandoned, and that they write their contribution on the nurses' notes!)
2. Breaking bad news should be the task of whoever is able to relate to the patient, irrespective of discipline. In many cases this was the nurse, but not exclusively so.
3. Having to 'find the right nurse' was still seen as a problem, but reverting back to the doctor relating only to a nurse-in-charge was seen as something that helped doctors, not patients, and it was agreed that the doctors would either have to tolerate the inconvenience, or arrange to come at a set time so that the nurses could plan to be available.
4. Leadership of the team related to the patient's primary needs. In a setting like the Burford unit, the doctor was not the natural leader of the team.
5. Team conflict directly affects patient care.
6. The lay voice expressed through the patient simulators suggested that the basic ideas being toyed with in the unit matched the needs of patients.

CONSOLIDATING THE CHANGES

After four and a half months, the changes had become practice norms, with little evidence of staff regressing back to the previous working styles. The medical staff increasingly related to the primary nurses, and the paramedical staff acted largely as consultants. However, it was evident that the change programme had demanded a high energy input from nurses and care assistants, and there was a general reluctance to pursue the evaluation phase as staff felt it would throw up further needs for change, and thus, further investment of energy. These feelings were attenuated when attention was paid to the unit by the national nursing press; the unit's name was changed in recognition of its changes in the nature of nursing work; and a teaching role to others was adopted. The 'fame explosion' in the nursing press arose out of no less than eighteen articles, including three cover stories, in four different publications, and served to reinforce the staff's views that what had been changed was worth it. The unit was previously known as Burford Cottage Hospital, and the authorities redesignated it as 'Burford Community Hospital and Nursing Development Unit'. All of the post-basic nursing courses were to be seconded to the unit to see 'its radical approaches' and numerous requests for opportunities to visit it were received from nurses and doctors from the United Kingdom and overseas. All of these developments appeared to alleviate the previously apparent reluctance of the staff to pursue evaluation and further change.

By the end of this phase, all of the action plan had been implemented, and was generally well accepted by staff and consumers.

8 Evaluating the changes

As the new norms became established, and a data-base was accrued from the action-taking process, I gradually withdrew from active clinical work to enable the staff to take control of the work. This withdrawal from being a full member of the workforce marked the beginning of the evaluation phase of the action research process. For over two years, I had contributed to the 'real' nursing work, and this allowed me to hold honorary full membership of the staff group and maintain a participant observer stance, while not fully participating in work.

Evaluation in the Susman and Evered (1978) model serves four functions:

1. Its first function is to change the place of study in reality by evaluating the effectiveness and feasibility of pursuing those changes generated through the action research process.
2. It is concerned with evaluating the diagnostic, planning and action-taking phase in the context of a research exercise which aims at generating new knowledge or theory. Its second function is to generate knowledge which can be used in other similar areas.
3. It verifies any hypotheses which arise from the study.
4. It provides the basis for deciding the next steps to be taken (Friedrichs, 1979).

Susman and Evered (1978) state that:

> We believe that most of our significant knowledge about social systems has grown by conjecturing.... Consistent with an action mode of inquiry, we often test out the consequences of our conjectures by taking actions and either strengthen or weaken our belief in such conjectures as a result.

It was assumed at the beginning of the study that all four functions could be worked towards by attempting to test out the consequences of the action taken in Burford Hospital in three ways:

1. To compare the quantifiable findings of the patient, nurses, and ancillary surveys and the findings of Qualpacs assessments; with a repeat of these measures to be conducted in the evaluation phase.
2. To compare the qualitative data collected in phase 1 with similar data collected in phase 4.
3. To analyse qualitative data collected as a participant observer in phase 4 in an attempt to establish the staff's feelings about the success or failure of the changes made in the norms of nursing work.

PHASE 4: REPEATING BASE-LINE MEASURES

Quantifiable measures

During the first four weeks of the evaluation phase, the patient survey, staff survey and Qualpacs assessments were carried out, in the same way as in phase 1.

The staff questionnaire was sent, via the internal mail, with an accompanying letter from me to the ten qualified nurses and the nine care assistants. Respondents were asked to return completed questionnaires directly to me, and not, as in phase 1, to the senior nursing officer, since, with the reorganisation of the National Health Service, the senior nursing officer post has ceased to exist. It was hoped that this difference in procedure would not have any effect on responses. The whole of the questionnaire was given to the qualified nurses, and only section V to the care assistants.

Two hundred people, selected randomly from the local general practice list, were sent the consumer questionnaire. An accompanying letter, similar to that of phase 1, was enclosed with the questionnaire, and a stamped addressed envelope was included.

Quality of patient care assessment: results

As a result of the use of this scale in phase 1 of the study, the method had become known to the health district, and a team of assessors had been trained to use it throughout the district by trainers from outside Burford Hospital. The two nurses who completed the assessment in phase 1 were asked to carry out a repeat assessment for four hours on a morning shift with typical staffing levels. In addition, four pairs of assessors from the district health authority group were also asked to conduct an assessment each for a two-hour period at any time during the day, with typical staffing levels present.

The five pairs of assessors did not visit the hospital before the assessments, all of which took place in the morning. On the day of assessment, the assessors selected the patients to be observed and completed the assessment as non-participant observers.

QUESTIONNAIRES

Nurses

All of the nurses completed and returned the questionnaire, and the data was analysed manually.

Of the five most important activities, three related to psychosocial care and two to physical/medical. Of the five least important activities, three were physical/medical and two psychosocial. It appeared that the qualified nurses saw information-giving, explaining procedures and allowing the patient to express her or himself as the three most important nursing acts, but that psychosocial care related to spiritual matters or to the patient's relatives were not of high priority.

Nine of the ten respondents subscribed to a nursing journal, with three of these subscribing to two or more. All respondents said they read at least one journal regularly. In addition to subscribing to journals, all read journals provided by Burford Hospital and four read journals received by friends.

All reported that they had been sent on at least one in-service course run by the Burford Hospital, and four said they had been sent on courses outside the hospital. All four had attended two outside courses, which consisted of:

- Holistic nursing (two respondents)
- Leg ulcer care
- Counselling research in nursing
- Family planning certificate
- Geriatric nursing (two respondents)

Seven had attended courses out of choice, but with the support of the hospital, in the following areas:

- Open University course P553 (four respondents)
- Holistic nursing
- Counselling
- Part-time MA course – Sociological research in health care

Nine respondents (90 per cent) were members of a professional organisation, and four of these had attended at least one branch meeting in the past year. Nine intended to stay in the same job for the foreseeable future, but two of these wished to undertake further study while working in the unit, and four hoped to progress. One respondent hoped to change jobs in 'a year or two'. Two nurses had each had three articles published in the past year. Eight nurses listed two or more articles or books read in the past year which were relevant to their work, and two did not. Seven were members of at least one voluntary organisation or activity group, and the following groups were mentioned:

- School committee
- Charity thrift shop
- Ladies Circle (Rotary Club)
- SSAFFA
- St John Ambulance
- Local Labour Party

- Anorexia Aid
- Village hall committee
- Wives club
- Flower club
- Local Liberals
- Local peace group

Questions in section III were designed to elicit the degree to which the respondent would assert herself in a situation, and how reasoned the reaction would be. Answers to each question were listed together and categorised:

1. This vignette concerned an error in payment of salary, with no forthcoming explanation. Seven respondents said they would immediately pursue the matter further, and three said they would insist on an immediate answer being given. Three were thus prepared to assert themselves strongly, and the remaining respondents were prepared to assert themselves immediately.

2. The vignette concerned a request that the respondent see the divisional nursing officer, at a time that would conflict with a previous arrangement made to meet a friend. Four of the responses were to cancel the meeting with the friend, but three of these added that they felt angry about having to do so. Six said they would go ahead with the meeting with the friend. The majority were therefore willing to assert themselves in relation ot the nursing hierarchy.

3. The doctor discharging a patient home when the nurse felt it was wrong to do so was the subject of this vignette. All respondents said that the issue was one that demanded agreement of the nurse, and indicated that they would not go ahead with the discharge despite the doctor's view.

4. This vignette involved being pushed out of the bus queue. Six said they would explain the situation to the conductor and hope he would act accordingly; three said they would wait for the next bus; and one she would get on the bus and refuse to get off.

5. The final vignette in this section concerned another nursing colleague at work who asked the respondent to admit a patient whilst she 'did the pharmacy'. All said they would refuse to admit the patient and suggest to the colleague that the pharmacy could wait.

The results broadly suggest a fairly assertive group of nurses, who were prepared to challenge both peers and superiors in issues which they felt strongly about.

The fourth section was designed to assess empathy levels, using the empathy rating scales developed by Carkhuff (1969). Two of the respondents received scores indicative of low empathetic functioning, and eight received scores which suggested high empathetic ability.

The answers to the ten sentence completion questions in section V were categorised by an external judge, and the results suggested that all the qualified nurses saw their role as one that focused on 'care' with all (n = 10) responding in this way. The 'good nurse' was seen to be either caring (10 per cent, n = 3) or being able to meet patients' needs (70 per cent), and the 'poor nurse' was seen as uncaring or as someone unable to think about the patient's feelings. All felt that nurses need a good general education. The majority liked the hospital's size and closeness to the community, and disliked the available facilities.

Care assistants

All of the care assistants returned the questionnaire (n = 9), which consisted of the sentence completion questions which comprised section V of the qualified nurses' questionnaire. The results were analysed manually.

The untrained workers appeared to hold some similar views to the qualifed staff, but a number of differences were apparent. Three (33 per cent) felt that nurses needed to 'keep up to date' educationally, whereas none of the nurses felt this, and 44 per cent of the care assistants thought that the best thing about the hospital was its 'friendly atmosphere', with none of the nurses responding in such a way. The nurses were unanimous in saying that the facilities were the worst aspect of the hospital, but only 23 per cent of the care assistants said this. Sixty-six per cent of them criticised other aspects such as 'poor wages for care assistants' and the 'lack of routine'. While the nurses saw the difference between Burford Hospital and the larger general hospital as lying in the role of the nurse and in its closeness to the community, the majority of the care assistants (89 per cent, n = 8) saw the latter as the most distinguishing difference.

Consumers

Consumers returned 121 questionnaires, giving a response rate of 60.5 per cent. Two were accompanied by a letter, criticising the questionnaire design. The sample characteristics are shown in Table 8.1. Sixty-three per cent (n = 76) were female, and 30.5 per cent (n = 37) were over 65. Forty respondents (33 per cent) were from social class 3 (skilled workers).

The answer to the ten open-ended questions were all listed by question on a sheet of paper for each question and an independent judge was asked to place them in the categories established in the analysis of the consumer survey carried out in phase 1 of the study.

Table 8.1 Consumer survey – Sample characteristics: Phase 4

Age (years)	Number (n = 121)	% of total
under 25	13	10.7
26–35	21	17.3
36–50	22	18.2
51–65	28	23.3
66+	37	30.5
		37.2
Sex		
Male	45	37.2
Female	76	62.8
Social class (according to Registrar General's classification)		
Professional (1)	11	9.0
Executive/ Management (2)	22	18.2
Skilled (3)	40	33.0
Semi-skilled (4)	29	24.0
Unskilled (5)	19	15.8

The results suggest that the community saw the good nurse as soneone who is caring, cheerful, competent and patient, and who needed a basic education (35.7 per cent), nurse training (25 per cent) or higher education (20.9 per cent). While 24.2 per cent saw the work of the nurse as carrying out doctors' orders, 75.8 per cent did not, with 30 per cent seeing it as giving care, and 25 per cent as meeting patient needs. One hundred and six respondents felt that nursing should be taught by a nurse (89.8per cent).

Forty-five per cent (n = 54) thought that convenience and closeness was the hospital's greatest advantage, and 18.3 per cent (n = 22), the quality of care. No one cited friendliness or homely atmosphere as the best characteristic. The worst aspect of the hospital was its small size (25.5 per cent, n = 25) and only 4 (4.1 per cent) mentioned threat of closure. The difference between Burford Hospital and a larger hospital were mainly related to a more personal service (40 per cent), more responsibility placed on the nurse (19.2 per cent) and the large proportion of elderly patients.

The results suggested that the local population saw Burford Hospital as a useful, handy and high-quality service, and that nursing within it was concerned with caring and demanded more responsibility from nurses than other hospitals.

QUALITY OF CARE ASSESSMENT

A total of five separate assessments were carried out over a period of three weeks and involved 10 assessors (two for each assessment). All of the assessors were nurses who had no involvement in the work of the Burford hospital. The overall results are shown in Table 8.2. The mean overall score for all assessments was 4.1, which indicates above the 'good level of practice.

Table 8.2   Mean Qualpacs scores

Assessment no.	Psycho-social individual	Psycho-social group	Physical	General	Commun.	Prof.	Mean
1	4.5	4.4	3.8	4.3	3.8	3.9	4.1
2	4.4	4.2	4.0	4.0	3.8	3.6	4.1
3	4.5	4.6	3.7	4.6	3.8	3.9	4.0
4	4.2	4.5	3.7	4.3	3.9	4.0	4.3
5	4.9	4.3	3.8	4.3	3.7	4.1	4.0
Total mean scores	4.5	4.4	3.8	4.3	3.8	3.9	4.1

QUALITATIVE MEASURES

In this phase, I became more detached from the actual work, and it became possible for me to make longer, more detailed entries into the daily diary. Such data related to conversations between individual members of staff, groups of staff and myself, and observations in the ward. As in phase 1, data were recorded in narrative form and inferences were made. Analysis consisted of categorising the data through writing each on a card and grouping them according to similarity.

The results were that 194 individual observation points and corresponding inferences were collected and sorted into six categories, corresponding with those in phase 1.

THE NORMS OF WORK IN PHASE 4

Organising and delivering care

The hospital was divided into three functional areas, each running independently yet closely related. The day hospital, open five days a week, had its own staff of one nurse and one care assistant, and the minor casualty area was staffed with a nurse who worked there exclusively from 9 am to 4 pm, Monday to Friday. Outside these hours, a ward nurse would have to attend to any casualty patients. The observations were limited to the care of in-patients only. The work pattern established in the action-taking phase had been developed and changed according to the individual patients in the ward, and a variety of other factors. For example, on cold, dark mornings, patients tended to sleep until 8 or 9 am, while on brighter days, some woke and got up as early as 5.30 am.

Between 8 am and 5 pm, two nurses and two care assistants were on duty, and between 5 pm and 8 am, one nurse and one care assistant. During the 8–5 shift, each nurse was responsible for a specific group of patients and gave all direct care. On the other shifts, the nurse was responsible for giving direct care to all patients. Care assistants spent most of their time on domestic duties such as cleaning, filling water jugs, washing up, etc. but were also often involved in either assisting the nurse or in getting things ready for her. For example:

> Primary nurse 1 is washing Mr A and dressing him on the bed. He is very big, helpless and heavy. Care assistant 1 is cleaning the bath in the bathroom leading off from the four-bed room. Primary nurse 1 calls for the care assistant's help, and together, they get the almost fully dressed Mr A out of bed into the wheelchair, pulling up his trousers in the process. The nurse asks the care assistant to bring the electric razor, and asks for an enema tray to be got ready for Mrs B, who is the next patient to be attended. The care assistant gets the razor and tray, and goes back to cleaning the bath. The nurse finishes shaving Mr A, pushes him into the day room, and moves to Mrs B. The effect is of calm: the nurse never leaves the patient group for long, and she is always in sight. The care

assistant spends little time standing watching the nurse, but slowly and quietly focuses on a major task, and then leaving it, often to respond to the nurse's requests. Most of the time, both work alone, helping each other out when need be. Sitting in the ward in the middle of four helpless people, one nurse, and a care assistant who occasionally 'pops in', all seems remarkably relaxed and normal. It feels like a family who have no routine because they are learning to cope with something new to them, yet in tune enough with each other to avoid chaos.

Each shift change begins with one nurse handing over to the other coming on duty, at the patient's side. The care assistants are not included, but are briefed by the nurse about the pattern of the shift's work:

Primary nurse: OK, can you be with me this morning, Mary? Mr D is off home at about 10 and wants a bath now, so I'll give you a shout when Mr D is ready to get in the bath. You might as well get on with your own plans till then, because he'll probably want me to pack his things up before I get him into the bathroom.

The physical work was not usually finished by a specific time. Sometimes all the patients would be up and dressed, with the nurse sitting talking to them by 9.30 am. At other times, beds would be unmade, and some patients still in them at 1 pm. The telephone was answered by a volunteer from the community, and calls would be directed to the nurse responsible for the patient concerned. Similarly, if the doctor came, he would see the nurse caring for the patient. At 11.30 am, the two nurses and two care assistants usually had a cup of tea before 'dinners'. These were served to each patient by his or her own nurse, who would then give each patient who needed medication, their own medicine guide and tray of medicine bottles. The patient would then select the correct bottle, take the correct dose and the tray would be taken away. When the patients had finished this, one nurse would go for her lunch, and the other would do so on her return. At 2 pm both care assistants went off duty, leaving two nurses on duty from 2–5 pm. In the evening, again, no set routine was apparent, except that supper and medicines were given at 6 pm. Throughout the night, the scene was similar. Work was unhurried yet constant, in that the nurses and care assistant were always doing something, and nurses were often sitting with patients in the day room or at their bedside.

Patients

Sixty-seven patients were admitted during the observation period, 61 of whom were over 65 (91 per cent), and 58 over 75 (86 per cent). Seven of them were transferred from the District General Hospital, and the remainder were admitted directly from home. Of these 60 direct admissions, 32 (53 per cent) were arranged by nurses directly to relieve caring relatives, and 28 (47 per cent) were admitted for acute medical reasons such as stroke, pneumonia or carcinoma. Of these 28, 14 had been visited on referral to the hospital by one of the nurses prior to admission. Thus, all patients had been referred to a nurse, and 46 had been admitted with full nursing involvement. Discharge of patients was the responsibility of the primary nurse, in liaison with other professionals involved, e.g. the physio, doctor, etc.

The average length of stay was 14.5 days.

Patients were unanimous in their praise of the hospital and the care they received, although two did complain about the poor facilities (specifically, peeling paintwork and inadequate toilets). They frequently expressed feelings of gratitude towards nurses and doctors equally, and saw themselves as 'ill people' who needed both medicine and nursing:

'The doctor said he thought I could do with some nursing in here because the district nurse could only see me for half an hour a day. So the nurse came to see me and said that they could probably teach me how to walk better, and get the physio to advise them. Well, I was keen to try anything, so I said "yes". The doctor was right, as well. I'm much better now, thanks to him and the nurses. My nurse says I'm nearly as fit as her now. I wish I was! But still, I'm much better.'

The patient generally referred to 'my doctor' and 'my nurse', and could usually name their own nurse:

'Sheila — that's my nurse — rang my son to tell him I was admitted.'

And they indicated how much having their 'own' nurse helped them:

'In the District General Hospital, I used to dread getting up because I'd have to nearly fight with the nurses to get them to do it the way I find least painful. But with your own nurse, you see, she gets to know and she writes it on the plan there, and everybody follows it. But, more than that, really, it means you have one person who knows all about you, and you can get them to phone her if necessary. Let's say the doctor wants you to do something you know you can't do, and he doesn't believe you — your own nurse, or at least Brenda [patient's nurse], would put him right, and he'd listen because he knows she's your nurse.'

The nurses themselves were ambivalent about patients. One of the primary nurses saw them as old 'geriatrics' who did not need nursing. The majority, however, made little reference to age. They saw the patients as needing nursing because they needed help in becoming independent, or in coping with dependence. While the nurses felt that most patients did not need very much medical involvement, the patients still wanted to see the doctor and were disappointed if he did not visit regularly. This caused some resentment in some nurses:

> 'It really annoys me when they ask the doctor about going home, as if I had nothing to do with it.'

> 'She said to me "Hadn't you better ask doctor about it before I start using a stick?"' I said: "No it's OK", and she said: "Well, I don't want you to get into trouble." I really have to bite my tongue. She was really trying to be kind, but it gets me down when people here still don't see nurses as thinking people who are not the doctors' handmaidens. Still, I went and asked him, didn't I, to reassure her!'

Patients were pleased about the nurses becoming 'involved' with them, and only one mentioned that he would like to be 'more anonymous'.

The primary nurses overtly challenged detachment and entered into very difficult relationships. Mrs O, for example, was referred to the hospital by a GP from a neighbouring practice for 'good psychosocial nursing' which, he said, could only be found there. She was 35 years old, with two young children, and had terminal cancer. Mrs O was not able to accept the finality of her diagnosis and had sought treatment from a variety of medical and non-medical practitioners without success. She ignored her children and husband, and was withdrawn and apathetic. Psychiatric help had not been successful, and she and her family were unhappy and depressed.

The nurse allocated a primary carer to Mrs O became intensely involved in the situation, and sought much support from both me and the GP in coping with this. She was upset about a 35-year-old dying; angry about Mrs O's rejection of the children; and furious with Mrs O's refusal to try to accept her situation and do something pleasurable with the family. With support, the nurse developed an approach of total honesty with Mrs O. When the nurse felt angry, she said so, and explained why to the patient; she spent a period each day with Mr O, Mrs O and the children together; she came to know the husband's worries, fears, angers and guilt; and she shed tears with Mrs O and her family often. Little changed in the situation, and Mrs O died without coming to terms with impending death or reconciling herself with her family. Afterwards, the nurse reflected on the involvement:

'It was so traumatic; I lived through that *with* them all, not alongside them. That's involvement, I suppose, and yet, it's true, it's much, much harder than being detached. But, God, it was so much more real and, I think, helpful. The husband and the doctor both praised the care to the hilt – and they meant it. That awful, dreadful few weeks with no happy ending, was, in fact, one of my big successes.'

Planning and evaluating care

All patients had a set of notes consisting of a nursing assessment sheet, a care plan sheet; progress notes sheets and lab results, etc. All disciplines used the same set of records, and these were kept at the patient's bedside and available to him or her. On admission, the primary nurse would build up, over a period of one to three days, an assessment of the patient's abilities and limitations in the twelve activities of living. From this, the nurse and patient together would identify actual and potential problems, realistic goals to be achieved, and detailed plans of action to meet these goals. Progress was recorded by primary and associate nurses on the progress notes. Doctors, physios, etc. also recorded their assessments on the notes, and their plans were incorporated into the care plan. Subjective analysis of the notes revealed an emphasis on physical care, but inclusion, in most, of psychosocial needs. Many patients did not read their own notes:

'No, I never bother looking at them. Sue always tells me what's going on anyway.'

'I can look at them if I want to, but I don't – because I don't want to.'

Some, however, did read them meticulously:

'I like to look at them every day; mainly because they are there, I suppose.'

'Of course I do. I've been in hospital so many times (more than half my life if you added it up) and I've always thought that I should have the right to see what they are saying about me. So, I've got the chance here and I use it. No other place gives you that right, and if nobody read them here, they might say it's unnecessary and stop it. In point of fact, you're told absolutely everything here, and don't really need to see your notes. But I think being able to see them actually encourages the nurses to include you in everything. The doctors, though, forget we can read them, and probably write things they haven't told you. But I can't read my doctor's writing, so it's a bit of a waste of time with theirs.'

The nurses laid great importance on report writing, sitting at the patients' dining table in the afternoon to do so whenever they could.

Two of the three primary nurses felt strongly that the notes were important, and in sharing them with patients, whereas the third found it a chore and often failed to tell patients she was caring for about their freedom to read the notes. This was reflected in the quality of the notes, and in their use. The third nurse tended to have shorter, less specific care plans, less complete assessments than the other two and the doctors frequently read the notes of the other two nurses virtually automatically on visiting the patient, but usually failed to do so when seeing patients under the care of the third nurse. The other primary and associate nurses were often angry about the quality of these notes, but the nurse would improve for a day or two when told about this, then revert back to poor notes.

The multidisciplinary team

'The team' was a frequently used term by all members of it, and was well understood by many of the patients:

Researcher: Who decided you could go home tomorrow?
Patient: Well, I asked Brenda [primary nurse], and she said it was up to me but that she wasn't sure if it was wise for me to go yet. I said I'd take her advice, but she wanted to talk about it at the team meeting, so I agreed to that. So really, it was the team who decided.
Researcher: What sort of team is it?
Patient: Oh, it's just your nurse, your doctor, your district nurse, and then social workers and those sort of people.

All patients seemed to be seen as needing a team of people to help them, and the primary nurse was seen as the mediator between the patient and the rest of the team, and the co-ordinator of the team's activities for that particular patient. Doctors and nurses particularly like the idea of the team:

Doctor: Having the teams means many less major problems with the old ones − we seem to be able to cope much better now. For me, it also means that I no longer have to bear the brunt of everything. The team can take responsibility sometimes, instead of it always being just the doctor.
Nurse: Because we all know what each can offer, we value each other more. I think the patient benefits mainly because he doesn't just see a stream of different people asking the same questions. He sees a group of people working together and pooling expertise.

Although, on the whole, the team did seem to operate well, conflict still arose, particularly between doctors and other disciplines. On the one hand, the doctors said they were equal partners in the team, while on the other, they would make decisions unilaterally and fail to understand criticism from the other disciplines when they made them.

Mr G had just been admitted this morning from the District General Hospital. He has terminal cancer, discovered when operated on for abdominal pain. The District General Hospital's staff have not told him his diagnosis yet. Sheila, his primary nurse, has written up a fairly comprehensive assessment and care plan, and has, over the four hours he's been here, established a beginning relationship which she feels will need to be deepened before she can do any real work. The patient's own doctor is not attending, and Sheila asks one of the town GPs to provide medical cover. She explains Mr G's situation to the doctor, adding that she doesn't know him well yet. The doctor sits at the ward table to write up the patient's drug sheet while Sheila attends to the patient in the next room. The doctor goes to Mr G, draws the screen, and informs him that he has a terminal illness and will not get better. Mr G asks how long he has left, and the doctor says a matter of months. The doctor leaves the hospital and Sheila asks researcher to go to office:
'Did you hear that? He's told the patient he is dying − left him − and not mentioned one word to me. We call that teamwork!'

Such events occurred regularly, with the doctors seemingly failing to understand how this conflicted with team work. Relationships with the physiotherapist and social worker were good, and they too appeared to be perplexed by the medical attitude.

Hospital social worker: The GPs believe in consensus if they agree with the consensus decision. If they don't, they disregard it and make their own decision. On the whole they are better than most, though.

The Doctors

The doctors regarded the hospital as 'a nursing unit for patients who need nursing. Our job is to support the nurse when asked, and to refer patients. It works well and we are fully behind it'. They regarded the primary nurse as crucial, and grouped patients according to nurse, for example, 'Whose patient is Mr A?' would mean who was Mr A's primary nurse. They trusted and respected two of the primary nurses, and had little time for the third, but obviously the primary nurse system was now seen as normal and desirable. Because of their belief that the patients were primarily in the unit for nursing, the doctors made only brief visits to the wards, and spent most of their time in the casualty area when they were in the hospital, and said they now spent much less time in the hospital than in the past. This was viewed with mixed feelings by the nurses, who, while appreciating that they now had more control, missed seeing the doctors. Formal ward rounds did not take place. The doctor would seek out the nurse he wanted to see, discuss patients and go with the nurse to see those patients needing medical input.

The physiotherapist

The physiotherapist visited the ward on each of the three mornings she was on duty and asked the primary nurses if there were any patients they would like her to see. Having seen them, she would teach the nurse and patient together any exercises, and this would be written into the plan. The majority of physiotherapy was therefore performed by the patient and his or her nurse, following instruction from the physiotherapist, and only specialised treatments such as ultrasound or short wave treatment were ever given solely by the physio. Nurses, patients and physios seemed to like the system, although some patients did suggest that they would prefer to have a physiotherapist.

Mary has just been helped to walk with her caliper on and using a zimmer frame from her bed to the other ward and back by her nurse, an activity planned two-hourly on the even hour on the written plan. She is helped to sit in her armchair:

Researcher: How are you getting on?
Mary: Very slowly.
Researcher: How do you like it here?
Mary: Everybody's so kind, but I would like to be home. I like it here, but there's no place like home, is there?
Researcher: You like being at home?
Mary: Yes, but I don't know when I'll get back there.
Researcher: You're worried about getting home quickly?
Mary: Yes, I think I need more therapy. I only see her once a week, you know.
Researcher: What do you think she could do to help?
Mary: I need more practice in walking.
Researcher: Have you told her this?
Mary: Yes, but she said the nurses are walking me six times a day, and that this is the only therapy there is.
Researcher: Are the nurses walking you that often?
Mary: Oh yes, they are very good. But they aren't therapists, are they?

Social workers

The social worker attached to the hospital attended the fortnightly team meeting, as did the social worker employed by Social Services in the nearby town. Both related largely to individual primary patients, or to the doctors, nursing officer or district health visitor for new patients. They were seen as members of the hospital staff.

Primary nurse: I rang Nick [Social Services social worker] just now about Mrs D. I often ring him for a shoulder to cry on when I can't get through to a patient.

There's no real social problem as such with him. It's really just a personality clash between him and the son, so I didn't refer him to Margaret [hospital social worker]. But I've asked her to come and join me, him and the son to thrash it out over a cuppa. I think it is the only thing to do, and she agrees.

Health visitor

The health visitor was part of the hospital staff, she had her office there and the hierarchical links with the nursing officer and the health visitor had been dismantled. Again, she attended team meetings but she was also well integrated into the ward. She would often call in to see nurses or patients, and joined the staff at coffee time.

District nurse

Seven district nurses were now attached to the town practice, and at the hospital, and responsible to the hospital rather than to an external nursing officer for district nursing. They joined the hospital staff at break times and were often on the wards.

All of these members of staff were part of the hospital 'inside' team and related well to each other. No overt role conflict was evident. The doctors, however, were regarded as 'outsiders' in some ways, since they never joined staff for coffee or worked together as a team.

Multidisciplinary clinical team meeting

The meeting was attended fortnightly by the primary nurses, district nurses, doctors, social workers, home-help organiser, community occupational therapist, health visitor and physiotherapist. The chair rotated between each member, and the discussion was patient-centred. At the beginning of each meeting, the chairperson asked each member to give the name of patients/clients they wished to discuss.

The meeting was relied upon by all disciplines, and 'We'll discuss it at the next team meeting' was a frequent remark made to each member and to patients. Patients were not, however, invited to the meetings.

The nurses

The primary nurses were regarded as the key workers by the team, and felt this way themselves:

> 'The primary nurse, makes or breaks the effectiveness of the team.' (Doctor)

> 'I've never ever had a job where I've felt as though what I do is crucial, but being a primary nurse here makes me feel this way.' (Primary nurse)

They were accountable to the patient for nursing care, and to the nursing team for clear care planning.

The role of nursing was clearly seen to be in assessing patients and enabling them to become independent, and cure was not seen as a realistic goal for nursing. Some confusion existed, however, about how nursing could achieve this. One primary nurse preferred a directive approach, while the other two were more non-directive. The associate nurses who worked in the evenings were also non-directive, but the night-duty associates found the flexibility in waking up times difficult. They felt guilty about not commencing work at 6 am, and expecting the day nurses to 'do all the work when we've been sitting here doing nothing'. Overall, however, the nurses saw themselves as 'professional people who are accountable for nursing care to the patients and each other, and not to the doctor or nursing officer'.

All of the staff found the work stressful, and needed to consult with the nursing officer over issues which they found difficult to handle. For example:

> Night associate nurse wanted to see me at 8 am. A patient had threatened to report her because she had let another patient go out to the pub. She felt it was right to do so, but should she have got the doctor's permission? Primary nurse at lunch time says she is worried about a patient she sent home last week who has fallen over and needs to be re-admitted − did she do the wrong thing? The same primary nurse has rung me at home tonight to say that one of her patients has died. She told the relatives today that he was improving and is worried about it.

Although the nurses wanted to be able to make decisions, and were making defensible and thoughtful ones, they were unsure of how to live with them, and lacked confidence in justifying them.

COMPARING PHASE 1 AND PHASE 4 RESULTS

The quantifiable findings

Qualified nurses
The comparison of phase 1 and phase 4 findings for qualified nurses was carried out manually and without the application of statistical method, on the advice of a statistician, because of the small sample size.

Section 1
The ordering of nursing activities for each group are given in Table 8.3. In phase 1, four of the five highest rating activities were medical/physical in nature, while three of the lowest were psychosocial. In phase 4, however, three of the top were psychosocial. In both groups, giving information to relatives, conducting the doctor's ward round and providing spiritual care were ranked a low priority. In phase 1, giving information to the patient was ranked as least important, whereas in phase 4, it was third in importance. The comparison suggests a change in the nurses' perceptions of their role in regard to giving information to patients and allowing them to express their feelings, but there was little change in attitudes towards the other activities.

Table 8.3 Comparison of rank orderings of importance of nursing activities in phases 1 and 4.

Activity	Phase 1	Phase 4	Change
Giving medicines	1	4	↓3
Explain procedure to patient	2	2	0
Keep skin clean	3	5	↓2
Record observations	4	7	↓3
Provide toilet facilities	5	6	↓1
Allow patient to express worries/anxieties	6	1	↑5
Give information to relatives	7	8	↓1
Provide spiritual care	8	9	↓1
Do doctor's round	9	10	↓1
Give information to patient	10	3	↑7

Section 2
A comparison of the results for this section is given in Table 8.4. A marked difference is apparent between the two sets of results. Phase

4 results show that the majority subscribed to a nursing journal, had
attended courses in the last year, were members of a professional
organisation/trade union, could quote articles used in the past year
and were members of voluntary groups, whereas these activities were
rare when the phase 1 data were collected.

Table 8.4   Comparison of rank orderings of nursing activities in phases 1 and 4

	Phase 1 No	Phase 4 No
Subscribe to nursing journal	0	9
Read at least one journal per week	9	10
Sent on course/to conference in past year	0	10
Voluntarily attended course/conference in past year	0	7
Member of professional organsiation/trade union	0	9
Attended at least one branch meeting of professional organisation/trade union in past year	0	4
Had one or more papers published in past year	0	2
Listed at least one relevant article/book read in past year	4	8
Member of voluntary group(s)	2	8

Section 3
A comparison of the results for this section is given in Table 8.5.
There is little notable difference in apparent assertiveness related to
salary at work (question 1); towards peers (question 5); or in 'the man
in the street' (question 4). However, the results indicate a notable
change in behaviour towards senior nurse administrators and
doctors. At the beginning of the study all (n = 9) of the nurses were
not prepared to assert themselves towards the divisional nursing
officer, but 60 per cent (n = 6) were in phase 4. Similarly, some of the
nurses in phase 1 said they would defer to the doctor's decision to
discharge a patient despite their disagreement, whereas 10 per cent
(n = 1) said they would oppose the doctor in phase 4.

Section 4
A comparison of the results for this section is given in Table 8.6. At
the beginning of the study, 88.8% (n = 8) scored low on empathetic
functioning, whereas 80 per cent (n = 8) scored high in phase 4.

Section 5
A comparison of the results for this section show a much greater
consensus within the group in phase 4 than in phase 1. Total

Table 8.5 Comparison of assertive responses

	Phase 1				Phase 4			
	Assertive		Non-Assertive		Assertive		Non-Assertive	
Vignette	No.	%	No.	%	No.	%	No.	%
(a) (related to organisation)	9	100	0	0	10	100	0	0
3(b) (related to senior nurse administrator)	0	0	9	100	6	60	4	40
(c) (related to doctors)	1	11.1	8	88.9	10	100	0	0
(d) (related to 'man in the street')	7	77.8	2	22.2	7	70	3	30
(e) (related to peer)	9	100	0	0	10	100	0	0
Mean	5.2	57.78	3.2	42.2	8.6	86	1.4	14

agreement was expressed in answer in sentences (b), (e), (g) and (h), but this did not occur in phase 1. The second application of the questionnaire seems to suggest that the nurses focused more on the individual patient than before, with 70 per cent (n = 7) defining the good nurse as one who 'meets patients' needs', and 70 per cent seeing the bad nurse as one who 'does not think about the patient'. The results for these sentences in the first phase were more diffuse.

Table 8.6 Comparison of empathetic functioning scores
Mean score by vignette (maximum = 10)

Vignette	Phase 1	Phase 4
(a)	4	8
(b)	2	8
(c)	2	6
Mean empathetic score	2.6	7.3

Comparison of high and low empathetic functioning scores

	Phase 1		Phase 4	
	No.	%	No.	%
High (6 and above)	1	11.1	8	80
Low (5 and below)	8	88.9	2	20

Untrained staff

In the first phase, 50 per cent of the untrained staff suggested that the nurse should identify with the patient, but the last phase showed no such responses, with 78 per cent saying that the nurse should be caring. At the beginning of the study, 87.5 per cent saw the role of the nurse as carrying out the doctors' orders, but this had changed to 100 per cent of the care assistants indicating that the nurses' role was to 'care'. The worst things identified about the study hospital in phase 1 were poor facilities (50 per cent), 'all old people' and 'the domestics having to help nurses' (25 per cent). However, the complaint about having to help nurses was not mentioned in phase 4 results, with the majority of care assistants (66 per cent) addressing individual issues, such as poor salary, personal relationship difficulties and the colour of uniforms. The 'need for nursing' sentence completion changed from a majority defining it as a deficit in self-care (75 per cent) in phase 1 to 100 per cent agreement and it was 'to meet special needs', and 89 per cent said in phase 4 that the nurses' work at Burford Hospital differed from others because of the hospital's closeness to the community, while no one responded in this way in phase 1.

Consumers

Because of the large sample size, all of the data collected from consumers were analysed with the aid of a computer, using the Statistical Package for the Social Sciences (SPSS) Programme (Nie, 1975). The already categorised responses were numerically added and transferred to the SER data-base, which was the input medium for computation.

Frequency listing and general statistical information were requested and the chi-square test was used, where appropriate, with the aid of a statistician.

The interrelationship between all of the variables and the results were all tested for significant differences using cross-tabulation of the application of the chi-significance. The conventionally accepted level of significance is that of a probability of p, meaning that the result would occur by chance 5 times in 100. The level of significance specified for this analysis was therefore 0.05.

Results

Sample
Cross-tabulation and the application of the chi-square test showed no significant differences between the two groups in age, sex and social class distribution. There were also no significant differences between groups and the proportion who were receiving care at the study hospital; what care was being received; in past care received; and in care being received elsewhere.

Consumer answers to sentence completion

Each of the ten sentence completion items were cross-tabulated by group, and the chi-square test was applied. No significant differences were apparent between groups for the following items:

'When caring for patients, a nurse should always . . .'
'A good nurse is one who . . .'
'A poor nurse is one who . . .'
'The best thing about Burford Hospital is . . .'
'The worst thing about Burford Hospital is . . .'
'When someone is ill, he only needs a nurse if . . .'
'The work of a nurse at Burford Hospital is different from that in a big city hospital because . . .'
'The best person to teach a nurse his or her profession is probably . . .'

In response to 'Educationally, nurses need . . .', the majority of group 1 replied 'a basic education' (46.5 per cent, n = 64), and the remainder were fairly evenly spread over the other categories of replies. In group 2, however, although the largest group still said ' a basic education' (35.6 per cent, n = 41), 20.9 per cent (n = 24) said 'higher education', and 21.7 per cent (n = 25), nurse training. More than twice as many saw higher education as a necessity for nursing in group 2, than those in group 1. This was found to be significant at the 0.04 level, when the chi-square test was applied.

In group 1, 63.1 per cent (n = 94) saw the nurses' role as 'carrying out the doctors' orders, while only 24.2 per cent of those in group 2 responded in this way. This was highly significant with a probability of 0.001.

Effects of other variables on sentence completion responses were measured using cross-tabulation and application of the chi-square test.

All of the responses from both groups were analysed.

Effect of currently receiving care at study hospital on responses

No significant difference in response to the following sentence completion items was found between those who were currently receiving some form of care at the study hospital and those who were not:

'Nurses should always . . .'
'Educationally, nurses need . . .'
'A good nurse is . . .'
'A poor nurse is . . .'

'The best thing about the study hospital is ...'
'The work of the nurse in the study hospital is different ...'
'The best person to teach nursing is ...'

Those who were receiving care gave significantly different responses from those who were not, however, for the following sentence completion items:

'Doctors prescribe treatment, while nurses ...' ($p<0.01$)
'The worst thing about Burford Hospital is ...' ($p<0.003$)
'When ill, I only need a nurse if ...' ($p<0.041$)

Table 8.7 shows how those who were being cared for in some way at Burford Hospital were more likely to see the role of the nurse as caring, meeting needs, carrying out procedures or acts other than carrying out the doctor's order than those who were not currently receiving care.

Table 8.7 Effect of receiving current care on view of nursing role

	Respondents					
	Currently receiving care		**Not receiving care**		**Total**	
Role of nurse	No.	% of total	No.	% of total	No.	% of total
Do what doctor orders	15	30.6	108	49.1	123	45.7
Care	8	16.4	51	23.2	59	21.9
Meet needs	11	22.4	29	13.2	40	14.9
Carry out nursing procedures	7	14.2	11	5	18	6.7
Other	8	16.4	21	9.5	29	10.8
Total	49	100	220	100	269	100

$X^2 = 13.03896$ with four degrees of freedom $p<0.01$

Over 30 per cent of those having present care thought that the size and facilities of the hospital were its worst features, and 33.3 per cent (n = 13) listed other issues such as internal decoration, draughty waiting room, etc. None of them complained about equipment or food, but 20.5 per cent did about access and transport. Those not receiving care, however, were less concerned about facilities, access or transport, and focused on size and other issues.

Effects of having care at the study hospital in the past on responses
Past experience with the hospital had no significant effect on the following items:

'Educationally, nurses need ...'
'A poor nurse is ...'
'Doctors prescribe, while nurses ...'
'The best thing about the study hospital is ...'
'The worst thing about the study hospital is ...'
'When ill, I only need a nurse if ...'

However, it did affect responses to:

'A nurse should always ...' ($p < 0.01$)
'A good nurse is one who is ...' ($p < 0.009$)
'The nurse at the study hospital is different because ...' ($p < 0.001$)
'Nursing should be taught by ...' ($p < 0.002$)

Those who had had care at Burford Hospital tended to mention competence as a desirable characteristic of the nurse; time as less of a difference between larger hospitals; and the need for nursing to be taught by a nurse, more than those who had no past experience of the Burford Hospital.

Effect of currently having care at other hospitals on responses
Only four sentence completion items were unaffected by the respondent receiving care at other hospitals. These were:

'Educationally, nurses need ...'
'A good nurse is one who ...'
'The best thing about the study hospital is ...'
'The difference between study hospital nurse and other hospital nurse is ...'

Twenty-two per cent (n = 17) of those having other care saw competence as a desirable attribute of the nurse, compared with 9.5 per cent (n = 18) of those who were not. This was significant at the 0.022 level. They were also significantly more likely to say that the poor nurse 'should not be there' and less likely to define her as 'uncaring' that those who were not attending another hospital ($p = 0.012$). Fewer of those who attended elsewhere for care saw the nurses' role as carrying out doctors' orders, and more saw it as caring. Fewer saw the size of the hospital as its worst feature than the others, and more saw the need for nursing as being associated with medical needs and less with self-care needs than the others. Only 78 per cent of them said that a nurse should teach nursing compared with 92.4 per cent of the others.

Effect of gender on responses

Gender had a significant effect on only one of the items. Most of the females saw the most important attribute of a nurse to be either competence (15.1 per cent), patience (14 per cent) or to be caring (46.7 per cent), which together represented 75.8 per cent of the responses, whereas only 57.4 per cent of the males chose one of these three attributes (competence 9.9 per cent, patience 10.9 per cent, to be caring 36.6 per cent). The difference was found to be significant at the 0.006 level (Table 8.8).

No other significant effects related to gender were found.

Table 8.8   Effects of gender on the desirable attitude of nurses

Attitude	Male		Female		Total	
	No.	**%**	**No.**	**%**	**No.**	**%**
Cheerful	17	16.8	23	14.0	40	15.0
Competent	10	9.9	25	15.1	35	13.2
Patient	11	10.9	23	14.0	34	12.8
Caring	37	36.6	77	46.7	114	42.9
Polite	5	5.0	–	–	5	1.9
Common sense	3	3.0	–	–	3	1.1
Other	18	17.8	17	10.3	35	12.0
Total	101	100	165	100	266	100

Effect of age on responses

No signficant differences in responses were found between age groups in the following items:

'A poor nurse ...'
'Doctors diagnose while nurses ...'
'The worst thing about Burford Hospital is ...'
'When ill, I need a nurse if ...'
'The best person to teach a nurse is ...'

'Caring' was the most frequent response made in all age groups, but those who were 25 and under gave a high number of responses of 'cheerful' (20 per cent) and 'competent' (15 per cent). Those in the 26–35 age group frequently responded 'patience' (23.8 per cent) and 'cheerful' (19 per cent); those aged 36–56 frequently responded with 'patience' (19 per cent)and gave the highest response of 'caring' of all age groups (53.4 per cent); those aged 57–65 emphasised 'competence' (14.5 per cent), and other non-categorised attitudes (24.6 per cent), such as 'punctual', 'attractive', 'well-groomed', etc.; and those 66 years old and over gave the highest response rate of 'competence' of the groups (18.2 per cent). Competence was therefore of most importance to those under 25, and those over 57, while the two middle groups, that is the 26–56-year-olds, were more concerned about personal characteristics of cheerfulness and patience. The differences between age groups were significant at the 0.002 level.

The education needed by the nurse was perceived differently between age groups, with a significnace of <0.016. All groups most frequently responded 'a basic education'. The proportion of those who felt that higher education was needed fell consistently according to age group, with 30 per cent for those aged 25 and under indicating a need for higher education and 5.4 per cent of those aged 66 and over. The youngest age group gave no responses related to medical knowledge, and only 5 per cent mentioned nurse training. All of the other groups included some medically-related responses, and a higher proportion responded with nurse training than the youngest group.

The two middle age groups again gave significantly different response from the others, in defining the 'good' nurse. While competence was a frequent responses from those aged 25 and under (35 per cent), 57–65 (24.6 per cent) and 66 and over (22.4 per cent), those 26–35 and 36–56 rated this attribute much less (9.3 per cent and 11.9 per cent, respectively). This showed a significance of 0.01.

Burford Hospital's convenience and handiness was seen as its best feature by the highest proportion in all age groups, but over 54 per cent of those aged 36 and over gave this response compared with 34.6 per cent of the 25 and under, and 31.1 per cent of those aged 26–35. The under-25s more frequently referred to the hospital's small size and the quality of the care given than the other groups; only those aged 26–35 frequently mentioning personal attention. The differences between age groups was found to be significant at the 0.01 level. Those 25 and under also responded differently from those who were older in defining the difference between the nurse who worked in Burford Hospital and the nurse who worked in a large, central hospital. The majority said the difference lay in the degree of responsibility (26.2 per cent), whereas those aged 26 and over all most frequently referred to the personal approach possible at Burford Hospital.

Effect of social class on responses

The social class of the respondent was found to have a significant effect on all of the sentence completion items. The attitudes said to be most desirable in a nurse were usually either cheerfulness or a caring approach in respondents from social class 1, but caring was the most frequently mentioned attribute in the other social classes. The proportion of those from social class 5 who mentioned competence was almost twice that of the others ($p<0.004$). The proportion of those in social classes 1 and 2 who said that nurses needed higher education or nurse training was significantly higher than those in the other three classes, at the 0.0001 level. Social classes 1, 3, 4 and 5 saw the good nurse as one who was caring, dedicated or competent, but those in social class 2 did not regard competence as highly ($p<0.001$).

The responses to this item regarding the characteristic of the poor nurse differed significantly ($p<0.05$) between those in social class 1, who most frequently mention 'impatience', and the other classes, who most frequently mentioned 'uncaring', 'incompetent' or 'when job is not a vocation'. Those in social class 3 were more likely to see the role of the nurse involving the meeting of patient needs, and those in social classes 1 and 2 were less likely to see her role as one of carrying out the doctor's order ($p<0.02$). Those in social classes 4 and 5 regarded the hospital's small size as its best feature significantly more than the higher classes, at the 0.002 level. Those in social class 1 were significantly more critical of the hospital because of the food provided than those in other classes ($p<0.001$).

In social classes 1, 3, 4 and 5, the need for a nurse was largely seen to arise because of self-care deficiencies, but this was significantly less in social class 2, at the 0.015 level. Those in social classes 1 and 2 were significantly more likely to say that the work of the nurse in Burford Hospital differed from that in a large general hosptial because of increased responsibility that those in the lower social classes ($p<0.001$).

Finally, there was a significant difference between those in classes 1−3 and those in 4−5 on the question of who would be the best person to teach nursing ($p<0.005$), with more of those in the higher three classes saying the nurse tutor than those in the two lowest.

Differences in the effects of extraneous variables between groups

Although group 1 responses were significantly affected by the three factors of currently receiving care at Burford Hospital, experience of past care at Burford Hospital and social class, these did not appear to indicate a difference caused by the introduction of the new practice norms. Similarly, the effects of social class on group 2's responses had no apparent association with the new norms. The significant difference between those who had had experience of care at Burford Hospital and those who had not in group 2, in their perceptions of what constituted a need for nursing and of the nursing role, suggested some link with the introduction of the new practice norms. As Table 8.9 shows, more of those who were currently receiving care based on these norms saw the need for nursing to stem from the need of the patient to learn or to receive care, and fewer of them saw it as relating to medical treatment than those who were not receiving care. In group 1, however, the majority of all responses to this item rated teaching fairly low. In group 1, no significant difference between those who had and had not had past experience of care at Burford Hospital was found concerning the role of the nurse. In group 2, however, significantly fewer of those with past experience of care at the hospital saw nursing as 'carrying out the doctor's orders' than those with no experience.

Current and past experience of care at Burford Hospital when the new norms were adopted led to the consumer viewing nursing as a service in itself, rather than as an adjunct to medicine.

Table 8.9 Major differences in the effects of extraneous variables on responses between groups

Extraneous variable	Group 1	Group 2	Apparent difference between groups
Currently receiving care at Burford Hospital	None	More likely to see teaching as a patient need which could be met by nursing and less likely to see 'medical' needs synonomous with nursing needs. ($p = 0.02$)	The changed norms led patients who experienced them to see the need for nursing as teaching and caring rather than helping the doctor.
Received care at Burford Hospital in the past	None	Less likely to see the role of the nurse as 'carrying out the doctor's orders'. ($p = 0.02$)	The changed norms led patients who experienced them to see the role of the nurse to be caring, meeting individual needs and carrying out nursing procedures, and not as 'carrying out the doctor's orders'.

QUALPACS ASSESSMENTS

Qualpacs assessments for phases 1 and 4 were compared manually and without the application of any statistical tests, on the advice of a statistician. The comparisons are given in Table 8.10.

The Qualpacs instrument indicates the following interpretations of raw scores:

1 = poorest care
2 = between
3 = average care
4 = between
5 = best care

The level of care in phase 1 was found to lie between poor and average; however, this was the findings of one single assessment. The past four series of five assessments are more reliable, given that the raters were all different and that the scores overall and for sections were within a similar range. The mean of the series scores (4.1) indicates care between average and best care, and none of the section scores fell below 3.6. Because of the disparity in the number of assessments carried out in each phase, no conclusions were drawn. The improvement in quality as indicated by the scores was, however, noted.

Table 8.10 Comparison of Qualpacs scores in phases 1 and 4

	Phase 1 (one assessment) only)	Phase 4 (Means of the five assessments undertaken)
Psychosocial/individual	2.8	4.5
Psychosocial/group	2.2	4.4
Physical	2.9	3.8
General	2.5	4.3
Communications	2.7	3.8
Professional implications	2.0	3.9
Total overall mean score	2.8	4.1

A COMPARISON OF OLD AND NEW NORMS

Figure 8.1 outlines the major differences in the norms of the unit between phase 1 and phase 4.

Prior to action-taking, nursing care was given by anyone. It was routinised, included judgemental interpretation of patients to determine care and was task-oriented. Patients were passive, and medical power was absolute, though resented. Nurses saw patients as old and dirty and not in need of nursing. The nurses, domestics and auxiliaries were regarded as outsiders. Good nursing was detached from patients, cure-oriented and patients were 'owned' by doctors.

Fun was generated on the ward to stave off boredom and monotony.

The phase 4 data suggest that a new set of values had been adopted, and new norms had become institutionalised. The nurses' role was perceived as being equal to other workers, based on involvement and oriented towards the achievement of independence. The patient was less likely to be viewed as old and dirty, and he or she had the right to choose his or her daily living pattern and to be involved in care. Only the doctors were seen as outsiders, and the rest of the multidisciplinary clinical team were regarded as real members of staff. Doctors no longer ruled unquestionably, although they were still regarded as being in charge by patients, and they themselves often only paid lip-service to team work. However, 'ownership' of the patients still seemed apparent, but instead of the doctor owning the patient, this seemed to be a prerogative of the primary nurse. Fun was used more as a therapeutic activity for staff and patients, rather than just the staff. Nurses were apparently feeling more stressed.

Staff evaluation of the action-taking

No predetermined plan to elicit evaluative comments from the staff was carried out, although all staff from all disciplines made comments in the course of daily practice and dialogue.

Nurses

All three primary nurses felt that the unit and its work had been 'changed' and that the plans formulated in phase 2 had been implemented. Two felt that they had become practice norms, and that it would be both difficult to alter them and undesirable to do so. The third primary nurse concurred with this, but was less convinced that the new norms were all for the better:

'I'll go along with the new ways, and don't mind them. But I come to work to earn money, and nothing more. I was happier supervising the others and using a routine. But I do like having more of a say in things.'

Not only were all three prepared to teach other nurses about the new ideals, but two were also full of 'evangelical zest' to convert others!

All of the associate nurses were positive towards the new norms, but found them difficult to maintain:

'Being non-directive is right in theory, but in practice you feel less of a good nurse when you're not telling people what to do.'

'I still feel guilty going off without finishing the work.'

'I believe the changed way we work is absolutely right. I just find it

Phase 1 work norms	Phase 4 work Norms
Patients:	
Seen as old and dirty; not in need of professional nursing if not ill. Patients liked routine. Patients passive.	Seen as individuals who need help to become independent, and therefore in need of professional nursing, whether ill or not. Patients liked having 'own nurse'. Patients liked freedom to choose own routine, be involved in care, read own notes.
Nursing Care:	
Could be given by any worker, trained or untrained. Routinised and task-centred. Directive and protective. Unplanned, based on judgemental criteria.	Given only by nurses. Flexible, individualised. Non-directive. Systematically planned, attempted to be objective.
Doctors:	
Unquestioned leaders	Team work highly valued. Primary nurse seen as co-ordinator.
Admitted and discharged all patients	Doctor's leadership questioned when patient's problems not primary medical. Nurse co-ordinated team decisions to discharge. Nurse involved in decision to admit.
Physiotherapist:	
Gave all direct physiotherapy with little nursing involvement.	Physiotherapy taught to patient and nurse and incorporated into nursing plan.
Outside staff:	
All staff regarded as outsiders except nurses, auxiliaries, and domestics.	All staff regarded as insiders except doctors.
Ownership of patients:	
Patients 'owned' by doctors	Patients 'owned' by primary nurses.
Nurses:	
Goal = cure and getting through the work.	Goal = independent patients
Role = supervising untrained, operationalising doctor's orders.	Role = giving care
Accountable to doctor/nursing officer.	Accountable to patient and peer group
Nursing officer:	
Role = supervisor.	Role = consultant.

Figure 8.1 Comparison of major qualitative findings in phases 1 and 4

incredibly hard to do it because it goes against all I've been indoctrinated into.'

The nurses as a whole felt positive about the new norms:

'I like the "permission" part of the new ways. We have permission to be involved as much as we wish, remembering that we are as human as our patients. Permission to laugh and cry with our patients like we do with our own family. Permission to do home visits before discharge. To go to the funerals of our patients, and time off to do so.'

'I feel strongly now that the whole crux of nursing practice is becoming a close friend of the patient. For this to happen, you have to change the whole nurse – patient relationship and we do that now through primary nursing.'

'I think most people go into nursing for satisfaction. I have more of that now than I have ever had.

'I'll get a patient's wife phoning up just for a chat. ... She'll write me notes about laundering his underwear, because she knows I'm the one to look after all that ... I feel I'm helping a family now, not just wiping bottoms and giving injections. And they care for me as much as I care for them, if I've got a cold or a problem.'

'No, I don't find it a strain anymore. It was more of a strain before, swallowing hard in the sluice and coming out with a prim and proper face.'

'I haven't learnt to do things differently. It's more that I've now got the confidence to make decisions I wouldn't have made before. I'm not waiting for orders.'

'Now I do things because it suits a particular patient, not because it's some standard routine. I think more about what I'm doing, and wonder if it's the right thing, and if it isn't, is there another way? I feel committed and interested. I enjoy my work more than ever before. I'd hate to go back to the old way. It's all so new and interesting. I just wish I were a bit younger!'

'Before I didn't feel responsible for any particular patient's care. You knew certain people had to do certain things, but you didn't feel it was *your* responsibility. I'm much more involved now – much more as a *clinical* nurse.'

'Before, I'd never have been the one to do something different from the common herd. But now I can make decisions and argue for them.'

Care assistants

The attitudes towards the change differed between those care assistants who were previously domestics and those who were nursing auxiliaries. The domestics regarded their new role as an upgrading and felt that care was better, while the auxiliaries thought they had been downgraded and saw no changes in the standard of patient care. They also expressed the view that basic nursing was best carried out by auxiliaries:

'It was far better when we did the nursing and the staff nurses did the treatments and admin.'

'I came here to be a nurse, and now the staff do all the nursing and we just help.'

Those who were previously domestics felt that the flexibility of the patient's day disrupted order, and found the uncertainty of each day's work uncomfortable. The ex-auxiliaries expressed similar views, and both groups were doubtful about the merits of the more relaxed attitudes to work achievement. They all, however, felt that the changes had led to a more interesting unit and felt more involved in the general policy-making than before.

Doctors

The views of the doctors were ambivalent. They preferred relating to the primary nurses because they were more aware of patient needs than a 'matron or sister in charge', yet they wanted the primary nurses to be supervised; they preferred the new, informal atmosphere, yet wanted more discipline; they valued the contribution of nursing expertise in decision-making, yet felt that nurses were largely emotive, subjective and therefore narrow in their judgements; they liked the way nurses got close to patients, yet said that the nurses got 'too involved' with patients.

The three doctors from the town practice spent less time at the hospital, because the patients 'really need nursing, not medicine', and the two doctors from an adjoining practice, who were increasingly referring patients for admission, felt that the new nursing norms were more helpful to patients, more satisfying for nurses, and superior to the previous regime and to prevailing regimes in other hospitals. Direct questioning of the doctors on their opinion of the new norms elicited positive responses:

'The hospital is now a very valuable resource to us and to patients because nursing practice is now thoughtful and reasoned. I feel privileged to be included in what I see as a really important development of a new model of hospital care focusing on the merits of good nursing, not medicine.'

'It is now a satisfying, open and effective experience to be involved here.'

'The patients here don't need a high medical input; they need the nursing input.'

'The nurses now do their job differently. We get much better feedback because the patients always now have the same nurse responsible for them.'

Other staff

The data involving other staff were only collected at the multidisciplinary clinical team meetings, where the team themselves spontaneously evaluated the changes of a number of occasions. This group as a whole was positive about the new norms, but frequently suggested that further changes would always be needed, and agreed on specific changes to be pursued. For example, an addition to the record system was made when the group agreed that the new system was better than the old, but would be even better with this modification.

EVALUATIVE CONCLUSIONS

The comparison of both the qualitative data and the staff and consumer survey data from phases 1 and 4 suggested that many of the new norms planned for had been incorporated into practice; that this had led to changes in perception of the nurses' role by staff and consumers; and that the new norms were generally thought to be better than the old by the staff. The qualitative data also suggested that the process of change used had a degree of success as a strategy, and that it involved education before change, active participation of all involved, and introducing a package of changes at one time, rather than gradually. The data did not, however, give any indication on whether or not the new norms had a positive effect on patients subjected to them. It was felt that the action taken could not be fully evaluated without an attempt to measure directly these effects on patients.

In relation to Susman and Evered's (1978) evaluation phase in the action research process as described at the beginning of this chapter, the data collected were seen to be appropriate to achieve their objectives. The function of evaluation is described in four-dimensional terms.

Both the qualitative and survey data appeared to be able to fulfil the objective of establishing new norms. The quantitative and survey data appeared to be able to verify the hypotheses that arose, and the change process itself identified the need to measure the effects of the new norms on those who were recipients of care.

The evaluative data were discussed at three meetings with the primary nurses, the health authority's senior nurse managers responsible for Burford Hospital, and a meeting of the steering groups set up to assist in determining the future development of the hospital's activities. At this stage, the changed norms had become known to the national professional press, and an 'explosion of fame' occurred over a six-month period, with eighteen articles written by journalists appearing in nursing, medical and health service journals, and the local press. Although the evaluative data had been analysed, conclusions had not yet been fully arrived at. However, the consensus view of both groups was that the new norms focused on providing a service which was primarily nursing, and that such a service was different from other NHS institutions; was well accepted by all disciplines; was seen as an improvement by all disciplines; affected the general consumer's perception of the nursing role; and had the potential to be cost-effective.

9 Lessons learnt

The purpose of the work at Burford Hospital was to explore four major questions:

1. Could the changes currently being advocated by nursing's elite be implemented in an 'ordinary' unit?
2. What effect would the implementation of such changes have on the perceptions of both nurses and consumers?
3. What effect would such changes have on patient care?
4. What process could be pursued in attempting to introduce practice change?

Because Burford Hospital was small and therefore could only provide a small sample, no single measure was found to provide answers to any of the research questions. Examination of all the results does, however, give interesting, albeit incomplete, answers in an area that has received little attention by researchers.

The results from the nurses and untrained staff surveys, and the qualitative data collected during my participant observation, suggest that the changes demanded by adopting the 'new ideology of nursing' were all implemented, to a greater or lesser degree, at Burford Hospital.

The pre-change norms of Burford Hospital were based on the assumption by the staff that physical care and 'getting the work done' were of crucial importance. Untrained staff were deployed in carrying out many tasks related to physical care and qualified nurses supervised this alongside carrying out technical and administrative tasks. The nurses were not generally active in professional associations and read little. They were reluctant to assert themselves towards nurse managers or doctors, and rated low on empathetic functioning. Patients were regarded as passive recipients of care, which was organised according to a rigid routine. They were seen as belonging to a doctor. Nursing supported medicine, and constituted, with untrained staff, the 'inside' group of the hospital. Other professionals were perceived to be 'outsiders'. The doctors had little understanding of the nursing role, and felt that nurses needed to be led by a 'good matron' and the doctor.

Individual care planning was unnecessary because of the well-developed routine, and patients had little say in what should happen to them. Information giving was not a valued activity and was seen as the role of the doctor. Patients were regarded as 'dirty', incapable of making decisions for themselves, and 'unworthy' of nursing care because they were not necessarily ill. The 'outside' staff were often regarded as nuisances, with little appreciation of patient needs or of the difficulties involved in nursing. Untrained staff regarded themselves as the real nurses who cared for patients, and they gained satisfaction from this, whereas some of the nurses were dissatisfied with the work because of the predominance of elderly patients in the hospital and the absence of technical, medically-related work.

The post-change norms differed markedly in virtually all areas regarded as targets for change by advocates of the 'new ideology'. Burford Hospital became patient-centred, and focused on the interventions of nurses as the primary professional function. Patients were regarded as partners, rather than recipients, and were given information and full access to their own records. Nurse-to-nurse information exchange involved the patient, and individual care plans were written with the patient's involvement. Nurses valued psychosocial care above physical/medical care, and gave care entirely, only using the untrained staff to assist. They were more assertive towards managers and doctors, and scored high on the empathetic functioning tests. There was less of a feeling of patients being 'dirty' or 'different', and they were seen as often being capable of making their own decision. Doctors saw nursing as the central activity of the hospital, and this view was shared by the other members in the multidisciplinary team. All these disciplines were seen as part of the staff, with only the doctors on the 'outside', and the nurse still used them as consultants.

While the data derived from the staff survey only show trends which suggest that a significant change was taking place, the qualitative data overwhelmingly support this assumption.

Together, the two methods point to the conclusion that the changes advocated in nursing can be implemented in an 'ordinary' unit without recruiting new staff, or incurring any increase in revenue costs.

The staff and consumer surveys suggested that a number of effects arose from the implementation of the changes in both groups, and the qualitative data supports these quantitative findings.

NURSES AND CARE ASSISTANTS

Both the qualified nurses and the untrained staff had different perceptions of nursing work after change had been implemented. The nurses' survey results showed that nursing was perceived as an activity equal to that of other disciplines, and governed by the individual needs of patients. This contrasted with the results of the initial survey, which suggested that nurses saw their role as somewhat subservient, depending largely on the doctors' prescriptions. Giving psychosocial-oriented care and information were now perceived to be important parts of the nurses' role, and subsequently, a greater level of participation in continuing education and professional activity occurred. The post-change responses to the sentence-completion items and the qualitative work suggested that the qualified nurses' perceptions of the nurse and his or her role had changed towards a focus on seeing patients as individuals and away from the view that the core role of the nurse was to carry out the doctors' orders. Nurses were more assertive in their relationships with other disciplines, and actively pursued individualised care planning and patient involvement. *Nurses no longer saw their role as supervising others to give care, but saw it as actually giving care.*

Although the new norms were said to give the nurses much greater work satisfaction, at the same time, they created higher feelings of stress and uncertainty when decisions had to be made or when decisions were questioned. 'Ownership' of the patient was a much-criticised characteristic before the changes when it was vested in the doctors, but it still appeared to exist after the changes. Now, the primary nurse 'owned' the patient. *Thus, one form of imperialism appeared to have been replaced by another.*

The changes in norms had a similar effect in some areas on care assistants. For example, they too were less likely to see nursing as carrying out the doctors' orders, and more likely to value the patient as both an individual and as a psychosocial being. Work satisfaction, however, was lessened by the changes. Care assistants felt that they had lost their status as nurses, and seemed to resent the advent of qualified nurses giving care.

CONSUMERS

A number of trends were apparent in changes in the perception of nurses and their work. *Consumers were now more likely to see nurses at Burford Hospital as competent, responsible and concerned with deficits in self-care.* (These trends were not, however, statistically significant.) Consumers in the post-change survey saw a need for education beyond a basic level – i.e. nurse training or higher education – whereas the pre-change group saw a need for a basic education only. The differences between the pre- and post-change groups in response to their perception of the role of the nurse was highly significant at the 0.001 level. In the pre-change group, 63.1 per cent saw nursing as carrying out the doctor's orders, whereas only 24.1 per cent of those in the post-change group responded in this way.

The changes made appear to have had an effect on the local population's perception of the care provided by Burford Hospital, and of the role and position of the nurse in delivering this care. The perceptions of the hospital staff were also affected by the changes and resulted in the adoption of new norms.

The effects of the change were largely positive, except in the case of the care assistants. Nursing auxiliaries regraded as care assistants experienced a feeling of loss of status, and felt less satisfied than before.

Both the quantitative and qualitative data support the conclusion that the changes made led to staff valuing the patient and themselves more, and in a growing clarity of role and confidence in fulfilling it. The essential subjective caring component of nursing gained in status, with a corresponding fall in the obsession with the superior value of technical and medical tasks. The assumption that exposure of the consumer population to the new norms generated by the 'new ideology' advocated by current nursing leaders will alter public perception and therefore expectations, of hospital care and the importance of well-developed nurses is supported by the experience of Burford Hospital.

PATIENT CARE

The quality of patient care as judged by Qualpacs assessments rose from below average to almost excellent as a result of the changes taking place. Thus, they appeared to have a positive effect on the process. This was supported by the findings of the Nursing Audit Assessment carried out in phase 5, which also aimed at measuring the process of nursing. The record of patients cared for in Burford Hospital after the new norms had become established all achieved good or excellent scores, whereas only 34 per cent of those nursed in unit operating in the traditional way achieved such ratings.

The results of phase 5 also suggested that patients nursed in Burford Hospital were more independent, more satisfied with life and more satisfied with care than those nursed elsewhere. Satisfaction with care was significantly higher at the 0.02 level. Elderly patients suffering from a fracture of the hip also spent less time in hospital overall if they were transferred to Burford Hospital. The reverse was apparent in the younger group of patients who had undergone hysterectomy who tended to have a longer stay. This may have been because the emphasis on nursing encouraged staff to delay the discharge of patients who had a hysterectomy until they had come to terms with their emotional response to the procedure. Although the sample size was small in the phase 5 study, it is reasonable to conclude that the findings suggest that the changes had a positive effect on the outcome of patient care. The similarity between the findings of Qualpacs and Nursing Audit assessments, viewed alongside the data collected during the participant observation carried out in phase 4, strongly suggest that the new norms resulted in an improvement in the process of nursing experienced by patients.

INTRODUCING CHANGE

The qualitative data collected throughout the first four phases of the study generated a mass of information about the change process evolved, and gives some structure to what was essentially a previously unplanned series of developments. The conclusions drawn from the qualitative data are based both on my understanding of what happened and the meanings I ascribed to changes. The usefulness of the conclusions to others is dependent on their trust in my integrity and judgement. Thus, the conclusions to be drawn from this aspect of the study are presented with due acknowledgement to my inherent biases.

Scott (1979) argues that the findings of action research studies must include the researcher's view of the research experience and that the relationship between the researcher and client groups need to be described in the report because 'unless some idea is gained of the quality and character of this relationship then the research report cannot be judged'. Reports of studies which rely on participant observation can draw out valued conclusions to the reader of the report if 'the essence is of trust that [the researcher's] reporting is seen as fair and honest' (Scott, 1979).

Not only was I a change agent, but I was also employed as leader of Burford Hospital, and therefore possessed a legitimate and a recognised authority to institute practice change in nursing. Such a triangulation of roles fits neither the accepted literature on the nature of change agency, nor of action research. In both fields, the innovator or investigator is usually expected to invest in the innovation and investigation, and the 'official' leader of the client group, if one exists, would be regarded as the client. It is argued in nursing that people employed specifically to innovate change, or to research into the processes or outcomes of clinical innovation, are able to do so more effectively than those employed in organisational roles.

The study suggests, however, that my fulfilling the three roles of organisation man, change agent and researcher was appropriate, and in fact contributed to the success of the action plan becoming reality. The legitimate authority gave credence to the initial first steps in the change process, and an opportunity to become a participant observer involved in 'real' work, rather than 'working with' the staff in order to carry out research. Conversely, the organisational authority associated with nursing in the National Health Service is frequently a distancing factor because of its traditional hierarchical structure. Thus, the strategy demanded by the situation involved my becoming a deviant nurse leader through becoming a 'real' worker who participated in and accepted responsibility for the achievement of daily work goals. The effect was to achieve credibility as a useful person who 'did' rather than thought about or directed the 'doing' of others. The hospital staff as a whole, including paramedical workers and doctors, valued highly the ability to look after patients. They appeared to accept me because I had this ability, and, more importantly, I had demonstrated a willingness to do so. This would have been much more difficult if I had been either an external agent or performed the traditional nursing supervisor role. The emergence of the strength of this approach has led me to conclude that change agents can successfully adopt a kind of triangulated role which will be beneficial in helping the client group to innovate change.

The change process itself began with increasing the knowledge base of the nurses, and the feeding back of the base-line findings. Ottaway (1976) argues that change is best achieved by educating after its implementation because a 'felt need' for education and training arises. Such an approach would not have been tenable at Burford Hospital. The staff were loyal to tradition, and there was a marked desire by nurses to maintain the status quo. The power-holders at that time were the doctors, and they were not in agreement with the new ideology of nursing, and any change would have been doomed to failure without their overt support. Changes could not have taken place without a shared perception of the need to change. The intellectual merits of change became apparent to all concerned, and the nurses themselves became co-researchers and change agents themselves when the attitudinal difficulties arising from the need to develop their intellectual acceptance into practical applications became clearer. This essential shift only occurred after the experiential sessions involving the use of theatre took place. This appeared to be crucial in the planning and implementation phases of the process. It resulted in the participants seeing the changes as theirs, and demanding decision-making rights. However, the doctors' permission had to be sought and was elicited purely as a result of intellectual argument. The assessing and planning phases of the study leads to the conclusion that planning change in the unit developed from describing the current norms of the clients to them, and by raising their consciousness of possible improvements, supported by establishing trust in the group and exposing their attitudes through experiential learning. It also depended heavily on the permission of the power-holders.

The implementation plan was based upon introducing the whole gamut of changes in 'one fell swoop', in contrast with the current belief of change strategists that change implementation should be gradual. The group as a whole feared that such an approach would require increased energy over a long period, rather than a period of intense activity and energy investment for a shorter period. The plan also emphasised the involvement of all disciplines in the change effort, even though it was primarily concerned with nurses, and focused on the multidisciplinary team as a whole rather than just nurses. As the changes became norms, the sense in this approach became more and more apparent. Changing the norms of any occupational group must be the business of the whole team of disciplines involved. In the case of nursing, it would seem that the changes planned for and implemented not only led to an increase in the valuing of nursing *per se*, but also to a greater valuing of the multidisciplinary clinical team by nurses themselves.

The implementation of the plan was hampered by the failure to recognise the need to bring about attitudinal, as well as intellectual, acceptance of the need to change and of the ideological basis of the suggested changes in the doctors. The hospital staff implemented the change plan with relative ease, but became frustrated and despondent when the doctors paid lip-service to the idea of equality within the multidisciplinary clinical team, and immediately demonstrated their perceived superiority by making decisions or carrying out acts which had previously been agreed to be seen as those which should involve the patient and the nurse. It became apparent that shared experiential learning between nurses and doctors was needed, and the interdisciplinary series of workshops using theatre conducted in the implementation phase brought about some positive attitude change in doctors. It is reasonable to conclude that, although it is possible for nurses to change their own practice, they feel a need for support from doctors. Although a lack of support from doctors could in some cases actually sabotage the change, in many cases it would not stop the nurses from carrying on with the new norms. Nurses, however, found it difficult to do things that did not win approval from the medical staff. The effects of the interdisciplinary sessions also reaffirms the conclusion arrived at from the planning phase of the study where the use of theatre is effective in promoting attitude change.

Active evaluation of the changes by the client group as a whole was seen as important by all of its members, and led to the development of further targets for change, and to a degree of conceptualising that is unusual in nursing teams. The multidisciplinary clinical team saw that nursing in itself was therapeutic and held healing potential as opposed to curing possibilities. Such cause and effect theorising by the traditional 'worker bees' of the system was a direct result of involving the 'subjects' of the research to the level of them becoming 'co-researchers' and meant that the end of the cyclical action research process, specifying learning, became merely the precursor to further pursuit of change along the same cycle. Burford's staff did not slip into the complacency of feeling that the task had been completed, but began again to plan further exploration, namely, in testing specified learning in the phase 5 study, and to explore ways of overcoming the apparent increase in stress and anxiety expressed by nurses with the establishment of the new norms.

The process of change that emerged was based on raising consciousness of the need to change before planning change; involving all staff in decision-making about proposed changes; using theatre as a vehicle for experiential learning; introducing whole, rather than part, change; and involving all participants in evaluation. The four research questions appear to have been partly answered, and the currently advocated changes in nursing seem to be amenable to implementation in ordinary nursing units; they had a desirable effect on both nurses and consumers; they were less positive in their effect on untrained people; and they led to an improvement in both the process and outcomes of nursing care. Although the findings relate to one unit only, and cannot be conclusive even within those limits, it would seem that the changes which nursing leaders urge nurses to implement are worthy of pursuit, and that their application raises issues about the nature of nursing work, the role of the patient and the role of the nurse.

FUTURE DIRECTIONS

A diffusionist view

If the new ideology of nursing is, indeed, of benefit to both patients and nurses, then it is logical that the changes introduced at Burford

Hospital to make the ideological issues practice norms are worthy of introduction elsewhere. The change process followed, however, suggests that individuals who are committed to the democratic introduction of change, and with the necessary skills to carry this out, will be needed to work in units. Introducing new practice norms would then follow a path of diffusion, where competent and committed nurses would begin to create a felt need for change and work with people to transform the felt need into reality.

The multi-method, multi-data approach of the study raises broader issues than could be readily resolved by drawing on the findings. Changes *did* occur, and they appeared to be beneficial and practical. They occurred only because the power-holders within the institution allowed nurses to hold some power. They also produced higher levels of anxiety than those experienced in the pre-change era as well as a growth of dissatisfaction among untrained nurses. However, the positive effect on patients suggested that radically altered health service extending to the provision of units where nursing offered the primary therapeutic intervention may be a desirable path to tread.

Power

The changes nurses are urged to pursue are regarded by some as a means by which nursing can become more of a profession, and consequently are often labelled as bids for power. On a number of occasions during participant observation in this study, doctors suggested that perhaps the changes proposed were more of a vehicle for enhancing the status of nurses than to enhance the standard of care given to patients. The nurses also felt that they wished to pursue activities to help the patient, not their own status, and 'power' was perceived as undesirable and concerned with self-interest. In reality, power was possessed by the doctors. Although the new norms gave nurses enough power to make decisions with and about patients, this power was delegated power, nurses possessed it because the doctors gave them permission, and visitors to the unit, as well as senior managers and administrators, often asked if the 'doctors approved' or 'how on earth did you get the doctors to agree to that?'. The possession of power is presented as an undesirable trait by social commentators when discussing professionalisation. Roth (1974) sees professionalisation as the 'avoidance of accountability to the public, the manipulation of political power to promote monopoly control, and the restriction of services to create scarcities and increase costs'. This view is also taken by Carr-Saunders and Wilson (1933), who sees professionalisation as a means to achieve power and is unconcerned with the occupational member's own interest. Power corrupts, and power-seeking is distasteful. Tiffany (1977) argues that powerlessness also corrupts: 'In the excessive powerfulness of the few and the potent powerlessness of the many, oppression flourishes.'

Under the old regime, patients were patently powerless, and oppression of them was obvious. The hospital staff, who regarded themselves as 'insiders', felt powerless against the 'outside' staff, particularly the doctors. As gatekeepers to health service provision, doctors held oppressive power, yet regarded the nurses' apparent bid for a share in it as undesirable. The whole issue underlying the changes introduced at the hospital was one of power: power for the patient to make choices, the power of the nurse to support these choices in an appropriate way, and an equal distribution of power throughout the multidisciplinary clinical team so that the person with the appropriate expertise and relationship with the patient could take decisions with patients to achieve shared goals.

Power *per se*, Tiffany (1977) argues, is not inherently evil, and 'to *be* is to be able to experience power: to *be* is to be *powerful*' (Bhola, 1975). Patients need to possess power in order to be. The possession of power by the direct care-giving nurses led to patients possessing power because the choices they made were not subject to approval by doctors' and senior nurse managers' scrutiny of policy manuals. The nurse giving care had the power to give the patient power to choose. Such an approach conflicts with the sociological conception of a profession, yet equates with the aspirations of those nurses who advocate adoption of the new ideology, and seems to represent the advent of a new definition of profession. While traditional professions gain power by acquiring a body of knowledge, surrounding it with mystique and keeping it a 'secret' from the consumer, and the semi-professions appear to emulate this style, nursing seems to be aspiring to a 'professionalised' occupation which acquires a body of knowledge, actively disseminates it to the consumer by adopting the role of teacher, demystifies the mysterious, and encourages the recipient of the service to make choices. All of this should lead to a share of power for the patient, directly challenge elite health care workers and reduce oppression.

Burford Hospital appeared to have achieved more sharing of power and to have invested power in individuals irrespective of discipline, and included the recipients of the care process. However, as it occurred under the overt patronage of the doctors, it is possible for them to withdraw this support, and thus render the patients and staff powerless. Although there was no sign of this occurring, the prevailing organisational structure was such that the doctors had the position and status to withdraw support if they wished, and this structure reflects the current acceptance of the power of medicine and

its superiority over other health care occupations. The newly
established practice norms in Burford Hospital oppose those in the
majority of other NHS institutions, and are likely to be regarded with
distrust by policy-makers and doctors. The apparent benefits to
patients and the whole of the multidisciplinary clinical team may be
seen as less important than maintaining the status quo and protecting
well-worn and established professional relationships and those
individuals who occupy positions at the apex of their particular
occupational pyramid.

STRESS AND ANXIETY

Primary nurses experiences a notable increase in anxiety following the
changes, and this was related to making decisions, coping with
uncertainty and being assertive towards others on behalf of the
patient. Menzies (1960) argued that traditional, routinised,
depersonalised and hierarchical patterns of nursing management all
serve to act as social defence mechanisms against the anxiety inherent
in nursing ill and needy people. If this is accepted, it offers and
explanation for the increased anxiety levels found in the study, as
these defence mechanisms were systematically dismantled in the
change process. The logical development in such a situation would be
to reintroduce the old norms, or to develop an alternative defence
system for nurses to use. The first option would need to be one of
choice if it became evident that the new norms produced levels of
anxiety which were harmful to the nurse, and particularly if the net
gains in terms of the effects on patient care were minimal. These
nurses did not feel that the anxiety they experienced was too much to
take. Instead, they sought help to cope with it, and felt it was worth
attempting to do because of the benefits the new norms brought to
patients and to their own work satisfaction. The second option,
therefore, seems to be the one that warrants further examination. All
of the nurses had graduated from a traditional, hospital-based
programme, and had had little experience in autonomous decision-
making. Handling decision-making, coping with uncertainty and
being assertive do not form a feature of nursing training, which aims
largely to inculcate obedience and discourage deviance (Stein, 1978).
Although the staff development programme implemented in phase 1
of the study led to a wish to institute the new norms, and to a belief
in them, it appears to have failed to equip nurses with the ability to
cope with its resulting side-effects.

THE UNTRAINED NURSES

> The single most important commitment at the present time is to ensure
> that qualified nurses nurse patients. It is illogical to do otherwise. It is the
> whole point of professional training and ensuring professional
> competence, and yet the majority of patients are nursed in the nursing
> service by the totally untrained or those in training. (Pembrey, 1984)

The shift in who gives direct care was achieved in Burford Hospital
and appeared to have a beneficial effect on both patients and nurses.
It also achieved a standard sufficiently high to alter the status
afforded to nursing by doctors and other members of the
multidisciplinary clinical team. Its one undesirable effect was the
feeling of loss of status and satisfaction in the untrained workers.
Such a finding, although not surprising, is important to patients and
society in general. The bulk of direct care is given by untrained staff
throughout the United Kingdom and this was the case in Burford
Hospital prior to the adoption of new norms. Such a position
inevitably leads to the untrained person perceiving him or herself as a
nurse, and the gaining of much satisfaction through this acquisition
of 'honorary nurse' status. Furthermore, the untrained cost less than
the trained, and their widespread use is a means through which a
service can be provided against a backdrop of economic restraints.
The justification of such an approach lies in establishing whether or
not it is necessary to have qualified nurses nursing patients, or
whether it can be done equally well by the untrained with supervision
by the trained.

The limited empirical evidence related to this question suggests that
the untrained rely on lay knowledge in their activities, and appear to
value routine, order and a custodial approach (Coser, 1964; Miller
and Gwynne, 1972). As a result, patients are encouraged to become
dependent on the trained nurse, and the goals of work focus on
safeguarding and maintaining, rather than using care therapeutically
to promote growth and eventual independence (Alfano, 1971). The
study shows consistent trends, which suggest that the nursing of
patients by qualified nurses did help the patients to be more
independent, more satisfied with life and to return home sooner than
when care was delivered by a mixed team of trained and untrained. It
led to clearer lines of accountability and less fragmentation of care
because the qualified nurses were able to give total care after the
change, in contrast to the giving of 'basic' care by untrained nurses
and the giving of technical care by trained nurses, which had been a
feature of Burford Hospital's working pattern prior to the change.

Law (1984) comments on the need to involve nursing auxiliaries before introducing change, and it is well known that this category of worker is often the most serious obstacle to the change demanded by the new ideology of nursing. To continue using untrained personnel to care for vulnerable people may well be cheaper than using those who are trained for the purpose and may preserve the status quo, but the probability that using qualified nurses is actually more beneficial to patients must be confronted.

NURSING AS A THERAPEUTIC FORCE

The notion that the changes introduced led to practice norms which facilitated 'professional' nursing was supported by all of the data. Professional nursing is nursing based on appropriate knowledge, skills and attitudes, and practised within a structure that made individual accountability of the nurse to the patient explicit. The effects of this style of practice were both quantitatively and qualitatively beneficial. Improvement in quality was suggested by the Quality of Patient Care Scale Scores, the nursing audit scores, the life satisfaction scores and the satisfaction with care scores. Quantitatively, patients became less dependent and had shorter stays in an NHS bed, and hence the system is cost-effective. All of these advantages arose in a system which required minimal medical input – an input which is expensive and therefore not always cost-effective. Hall (1969) suggests that nursing has traditionally been seen as an activity that merely supports the therapy of others, and argues that it should be recognised that nursing in itself is therapeutic. The collective findings of the study strongly support the argument that good nursing helps people to recover or regain independence and is of much importance in influencing the perceptions of the need for nursing and the role of the nurse in those who plan health care services, and those who influence the social policy related to these issues.

While the discrete conclusions of the study are in themselves of interest, consideration of them as a whole to allow for generalisation can be used to generate policy changes by the diffusionist.

THE BURFORD HOSPITAL FINDINGS AND HEALTH SERVICE POLICY

If power can be shared in the health service, nurses would adopt the new norms and be helped to cope with the associated stress; untrained nurses could be directed to different roles which offered them reasonable levels of satisfaction; and nursing would be able to develop its therapeutic potential. In addition, the development of the role of nursing, based on 'nursing beds', would be advantageous to the National Health Service as a whole.

Hall (1964) argues that patients in biological crisis require admission to an acute hospital, with its focus on medicine, but that many patients would benefit by moving out of such an environment when the crisis is resolved. Henderson (1966) note how many patients who are admitted to medically-led hospitals often need nursing, yet the gatekeeper role is vested exclusively in the doctor. This study points to the need for an alternative provision for both of these types of patient. The elderly, dependent person who contracts a bed sore, or who needs to be looked after because daily living is inhibited due to an acute illness (which would normally be coped with at home by someone who is usually independent), needs admission to a unit that focuses on nursing. No such units currently exist in the National Health Service. Patients who have had a biological crisis resolved could benefit from early transfer to a unit focusing on nursing.

Two possibilities in establishing this type of provision with existing facilities and using existing facilities are apparent.

First, the number of patients currently occupying medically controlled beds could be nursed in beds controlled by those who nurse. Therefore, many acute beds could be redesignated acute nursing beds, and a nursing unit within each acute hospital could be established. Hall (1964), Henderson (1966), Alfano (1969) and Pearson (1983, 1984) all describe an eighty-bed nursing unit which operates in this way, and the longitudinal study by Hall *et al.* (1975) which evaluated this provision showed it to be very effective in terms of improved patient outcomes; marked reduction in costs compared to medically controlled wards; commendable observable practices and innovations; and overwhelming acceptance of the unit by both doctors and patients. Referrals to the unit were frequent and it was regarded as an important resource to the acute hospital. Such units in the National Health Service could be established in existing staffed wards, although the resistance to them, organisationally and professionally, is likely to be considerable.

A second possibility, and perhaps less difficult to achieve in the short term, is a reconsideration of the role of community and cottage hospitals. Cottage hospitals were established in the mid-1800s quite definitely to provide nursing, but from the beginning were controlled by doctors. McConaghey (1964) details their development, and notes that they are important to doctors who 'themselves have jealously guarded the privilege of being able to treat and nurse them in them their own patients'. Historically, these hospitals have been noted for their high standards of nursing and have relied on the nursing input, with short, daily visits to patients by general practitioners, in much the same way as they visit people at home. The need for medical care in these hospitals is, by their very nature, no different from the need of those who are ill at home. The crucial determining factor in admission is the need for nursing. Yet they have been, and still are known as, 'GP hospitals', and admitting rights are granted officially only to doctors.

Many cottage hospitals were closed in the 1970s in line with the policy towards centralising resources in large, district hospitals. However, innovatory work in the Oxford Region (Bennett, 1974) led to a re-examination of this policy and a commitment to the creation of community hospitals grew. The concept of community hospital embraced the view that they would cater for people who needed nursing: indeed, the need for a high level of medical care was seen as a factor which would not denote acceptability of the patient for community hospital care. Despite the acknowledgement that the role of the community hospital was care, and that the bulk of this need would be met by nurses, doctors were still seen as the gatekeepers and controllers. Rue (1974) says: 'If the general practitioner has suitable treatment facilities he can, with his team, provide local care for many patients as an alternative to district general hospital care'; and Vine (1974), in describing the role of the specialist doctor, suggests that it is to 'help and support the family doctors looking after the community hospital'. Although doctors are seen as the vital professional group in community hospitals, empirical studies suggest that they are only of limited importance, with Oddie *et al.* (1971) finding that doctors, on average, spent 27.4 minutes per day in the hospitals. Community or cottage hospitals are nursing units in embyro. They could be easily revitalised to provide very valuable resources to patients if the focus of practice was altered from one encompassing the medical model and its associated dominance of nurses and patients by doctors, to a model for nursing associated with nurses working with patients in a way which allows patients to make informed choices.

Such policy changes in the health service would not, this study suggests, be merely a means for the aggrandisement of nursing. They would improve both quality and cost-effectiveness within health care in general.

RECOMMENDATIONS

The nature of the study prompts recommendations on future research. Because the study field was small, generalisation of findings is difficult and uncertain, and similar projects, using a triangulation of methods in various settings to explore all of the research questions, are essential.

Despite the limitation of this study, the following recommendations can be made:

1. That the new ideology of nursing currently being advocated by nursing leaders should be supported and further evaluated.
2. That educational input should be high for nurses required to implement new norms.
3. That internal change agents with legitimate roles within the organisation should be used more widely in the National Health Service.
4. That nurses who have adopted new norms related to primary nursing and individualised care should have access to support services because of the high stress levels involved.
5. That long-term policy should aim at the phasing out of untrained staff caring for patients.
6. That pilot nursing units should be established within the National Health Service for post-crisis patients and they should be systematically evaluated.
7. That community hospitals should be regarded as acute nursing units, and the staff should be helped to adopt norms based on a model alternative to that for medicine.
8. That further, large-scale research is needed on:
    (a) the therapeutic effect of nursing;
    (b) fostering patient involvement and autonomy;
    (c) effective change strategies;
    (d) the use and effectiveness of theatre in attitude change;
    (e) on how to help nurses cope with the stress that arises when the hierarchical systems which help to avoid anxiety are dismantled.

Appendix I

Staff questionnaire

---

1. Please give your qualifications:

2. *Section I*

   Here is a list of things which nurses are expected to do in caring for patients. Would you please number each one from 1 – 10, in the order which is, in your opinion, of importance, with number 1 being the most important. For example, if you think doing the consultant's ward round is the most important, write number 1 in the box; if keeping the patients' skin clean and dry is the next important, write 2 in the box, and so on.

   Give information to the patient about his condition

   Give the correct medicines as prescribed by the doctor

   Keep the patients' skin clean and dry

   Ensure that the patients' relatives receive adequate information and advice

   Do the consultant's ward round

   Encourage the patient to express his worries and anxieties

   Provide the needed toilet facilities (e.g. bedpan)

   Accurately record the required observations (e.g. temperature)

   Establish what the patient himself prefers regarding spiritual care, and arranging for the visit of a clergyman if necessary

   Explain the reasons for any procedures which are to be carried out with the patient

3. *Section II*

   Please answer the following questions:

   (a) Do you subscribe to any nursing journals? If so, give details.
   (b) Do you read any nursing journals to which you do not subscribe? If so, please list them and say how you have access to them (e.g. read a friend's; read in the library, etc.).

(c)   Please list any conferences/short courses which you have attended at the request of your employer in the last year.

(d)   Please list any conferences/short courses which you have attended voluntarily during the last year (including those which your employer gave permission/leave for, but attendance was specifically requested by you).

(e)   Are you a member of any professional association? If so, please specify.

(f)   If you answered YES to question (e), do you ever attend their meetings, and if so, how often in the last year?

(g)   Have you ever had anything published in the nursing or other press, or are you currently submitting something? If so, please give details.

(h)   What are your future plans in regard to your work (e.g. stay in same post, take another course, etc.)?

(i)   Have you read any books or journal articles which you have found useful to your area of work in the last year? If so, please give details.

(j)   Are you a member of any voluntary groups? If so, please give details.

4.   *Section III*

Here is a list of some situations which you may face in your daily life. Underneath each one, please write what you would do. Think carefully before you answer, and try to state honestly what your usual reaction to such a situation would be:

(a)   You have recently received your payslip, and found that £40 has been deducted in addition to your usual deductions. The nursing officer is unable to explain why, and a telephone call to the finance office results in your being told that the local staff do not know about deductions, but the computer will have a good reason for deducting the extra £40. What do you do?

(b)   You have been asked to attend the divisional nursing officer's office for an interview at 4 o'clock in a few days' time. You have already made arrangements to meet a friend at 5 o'clock on that day, and hope that your interview finishes in time to meet her. On the day of the interview, you arrive at 3.55, and meet a colleague outside the divisional nursing officer's room. Your colleague asks if she can 'pop in before you' as she only wants to see the divisional nursing officer for a couple of minutes. However, it is now 4.35 and your colleague is still in the office. You know that if you do not begin the interview soon, you will be very late for your planned meeting with your friend. What do you do?

(c)   One of the patients you are nursing is Mr Atkinson. He has had a CVA and has been in the ward for four weeks. He has gradually improved and, because of a great deal of work on your part, is able to get out of bed himself, dress himself apart from putting on his socks and shoes, and is mobile enough to get around the house. You feel that he will be able to put on his socks and shoes himself if he spends about one more week in the ward, and you continue to help and encourage him. Today, however, he has been seen by the doctor, who has said he can go home tomorrow. Mr Atkinson is unconcerned about whether he goes or stays, although he admits that it would be better if he could master full dressing before going home.

On taking this up with the doctor later, he brushes off your comment that you would prefer Mr Atkinson to stay, saying that he is 'taking up a bed without good reason, and it's a medical decision anyway'. What do you do?

(d) You are waiting at the bus stop, on your way home from work. There are seven people in the queue, and you are third from the front. As the bus stops, the conductor says that there is only room for three. As you begin to board the bus, the young girl behind you pushes in front. The conductor calls, 'That's all.' What do you do?

(e) You have had a busy day at work, and just as it is time for you to go off duty, a new patient is admitted. The nurse who is working the evening shift asks you to admit the patient and then organise the doctor, as she wants to finish ordering the pharmacy which she is in the middle of doing now. What do you do?

5. *Section IV*

Please write your response to the following statements in the same way as in section III.

(a) Mrs Tomkins is the ward domestic. She is usually very good, but lately has become somewhat slipshod in her work. Today, she has failed to refill the patient's water jugs, the morning coffee still hasn't come round for the patients and the kitchen is in a mess. It is 11 am and on trying to find Mrs Tomkins, you find her using the office telephone. When she finishes, you ask her what she is doing, and she tells you that she was ringing home to ask her husband if her eldest daughter (you know that she is 18 years old, and a bit of a problem) has come home yet, as she did not come home last night. What do you do?

(b) You are working in the casualty room when a patient arrives, having been seen in the doctor's surgery. She has, according to the note, fallen down the stairs. She is quite young, looks anxious and is covered in bruises on her arms, neck and face. You suspect that the bruises have been inflicted by someone, and in your conversation, she tells you that her husband has beaten her; this has happened a number of times; and you are the only person she has told. You want her to see the social worker, but she refuses, and sits down to tell you all about her husband's brutality. You eventually insist that you ring the social worker, but as you lift up the telephone, she shouts, almost hysterically at you, saying you have no right to telephone without her consent. What do you do?

(c)   David is seventeen, and is a disruptive influence on the ward. He has had a polyp removed from his ear, and is in the hospital because the wound has become infected. He insists on listening to the radio all day and the other patients, all a lot older than him, complain about the loud pop music. Today, you are very busy, and in the middle of the medicine round notice that he turned the radio up when you entered the ward. After the medicines you have some bed baths to do, and then two dressings, before the ward round. You are irritated with David, and when you tell him to turn the radio off, he does so and storms out of the ward into the day room. What do you do?

6.   *Section V*

Please complete the following unfinished sentences:

(a)   When caring for patients, a nurse should always ...
(b)   Educationally, nurses need ...
(c)   A good nurse is one who ...
(d)   A poor nurse is one who ...
(e)   Doctors find out what illness a patient has and prescribe the necessary medical treatment, while nurses ...
(f)   The best thing about ... Hospital is ...
(g)   The worst thing about ... Hospital is ...
(h)   When someone is ill, he only needs a nurse if ...
(i)   The work of a nurse at ... Hospital is different from that in a big city hospital because ...
(j)   The best person to teach a nurse her profession is probably ...

Thank you very much indeed for giving your time to fill in this questionnaire. Your contribution will be of much use in determining the maintenance of care in ...

Appendix II

Consumer questionnaire

Please complete the following unfinished sentences:

1. When caring for patients, a nurse should always . . .
2. Educationally, nurses need . . .
3. A good nurse is one who . . .
4. A poor nurse is one who . . .
5. Doctors find out what illness you have and prescribe the necessary treatment, while nurses . . .
6. The best thing about . . . Hospital is . . .
7. The worst thing about . . . Hospital is . . .
8. When I am ill, I only need a nurse if . . .
9. The work of a nurse at . . . Hospital is different to that in a big city hospital because . . .
10. The best person to teach a nurse his/her profession is probably . . .

Please answer the following questions:

11. Do you at present regularly attend . . . Hospital for treatment? If so, please give details.
12. Have you ever used the services of . . . Hospital? If so, please give details.
13. Are you attending any other hospital for treatment that you feel could be given at . . .? If so, please give details.
14. What is your sex?* Male . . .   Female . . .
15. What is your age?* Under 25   . . .
                       26 – 35   . . .
                       36 – 50   . . .
                       51 – 65   . . .
                       66 or over   . . .
16. What is your occupation? (If retired, please state occupation before retirement.)
17. What is your spouse's occupation (if applicable)?
    Thank you for your help.

*Tick which is appropriate.

Appendix III

Interview schedule – phase 5

Basic Biographical Schedule

Information to be taken from patient's notes

Initial patient history

Patient's name _____

Interviewer No. (i.e. 1, 2 or 3) _____

Date _____

Hospital no. _____

Patient's code no. _____

Menstrual status before operation

Menstruating	1
Menopausal	2
Post-menopausal	3
Non-applicable	4

Date of birth _____

Number of children _____

Sex _____   Male = 1   Female = 2   [ ] 15

Home tel. no. _____

Date of fracture _____

Diagnosis: Sub-cap   = 1   [ ] 16
             Cervical   = 2
             Inter-Trochanteric   = 3
             Sub-trochanteric   = 4
             Fibroids   = 5
             Prolapse   = 6
             Menorraghia   = 7
             Other   = 8

Date of operation _____

Operation   Thompsons prosthesis   = 1   [ ] 17
             Dynamic screw   = 2
             A.O. screw   = 3
             ABDO hysterectomy total = 4
             ABDO hysterectomy partial = 5
             Other   = 6

Consultant   _____ = 1   [ ] 18
             _____ = 2
             _____ = 3
             _____ = 4
             _____ = 5

Post-op Analgesia _____

Post-op recovery   [ ] 19
             uneventful   = 1
             complication   = 2

Inter-venous therapy
             yes   = 1   [ ] 20
             no   = 2

When mobilised (in days) _____

                                                [ ] 21
History of post-op confusion
             Yes   = 1
             No   = 2   [ ] 22

Group
     Ortho   Control 1   = 1   [ ] 23
             Control 2   = 2
             Exp.   = 3

     Gynae   Control 1   = 4
             Control 2   = 5
             Exp   = 6

Name

———————————————————, I would like to ask you
some questions about yourself, your family, and your social
activities. To begin with:

1. At the present time are you:

Married	1
Widowed	2
Divorced	3
Separated	4
Never married	5
Co-habiting	6
No information	7

23

2. Where were you living before you came to this hospital?

   Address ———————————————————————

3. What are the names of the other persons who lived with
   you at that address, how old are they and how are they
   related to you?

Name	Relationship	Age

24

25

26

(Code: 0 = alone, 1 = spouse, 2 = child, 3 = other relative
or friend)

4. Of those you have just mentioned or anyone else not
   living with you which one person:

   (a) Do you know best?
   (b) Spends the most time with you at home?
   (c) Will spend the most time with you after you leave
   hospital?

5. What type of residence did you live in before you were
   hospitalised?

		House	1
Part III accom.	5	Bungalow	2
Other	6	Flat	3
No information	7	Warden-controlled	4

27

6. Does your residence have?

Stairs	1
No stairs	2
Inside tiolet	3
Outside tiolet	4
Central heating	5
Coal or electric fire	6
No heating	7

☐ 28

☐ 29

☐ 30

Yes No
(1) (0)

7. Do you have to climb stairs to

Enter your residence	
Go to toilet	
Go to bed	

☐ 31

☐ 32

☐ 33

8. Where you employed at the time you were hospitalised?

Yes	
No	

☐ 34

9. When were you last employed?

Less than a year ago	1
1–4 years ago	2
5 or more years ago	3
Never worked	4
No information	5

☐ 35

10. What type of work did you do? (this includes running your home)

11. What is the highest grade you completed in school?

Secondary school	1
Grammar school	2
College/university	3
No information	4

☐ 36

Nursing Dependency Index

Patient
code number ☐☐☐☐

Date of
visit ☐☐☐☐☐☐

Number
of visit ☐☐

Day base . . . .

Interval since last
visit (in days) ☐☐

*See definition sheet performance of ADL activity	Independent	Independent with aids	Requires assistance of no more than one person	Requires assistance of no more than two persons	Bedfast	Activity score
Activity* Important note: Only score ONE performance per activity						
Score per activity	1	2	3	4	5	
1 Bed						
2 Dressing						
3 Walking						
4 Toileting						
5 Provision of meal						
6 Feeding						
7 Control of environment						
8 Washing and grooming						
9 Bathing or shower						
10 Chair						
11 Wheelchair						
12 Bladder function						
13 Bowel function						
14 Medication						
15 Treatment						
16 Management of household						
17 Emotional health						
18 Sleep						
19 Time up during day						
Performance Score						

Nursing Dependency Index: Professional Sources of Assistance

Patient code number ☐☐☐☐☐   Number of visit ☐☐

	Professional sources of assistance													
	GP	DNS	HV	MSW	ASW	HHS	MOW	VA	CH	DH	OT	PT	Res	Oth	Act score
1 Bed														
2 Dressing														
3 Walking														
4 Toileting														
5 Provision of meal														
6 Feeding														
7 Control of environment														
8 Washing and grooming														
9 Bath or shower														
10 Chair														
11 Wheelchair														
12 Bladder function														
13 Bowel function														
14 Medication														
15 Treatment														
16 Management of household														
17 Emotional health														
18 Sleep														
19 Time up during day														
Professional sources score														

Activities of Living Assessment

Nursing dependency score		
Total dependency requiring human assistance	39	40
	41	42
Bed		43
Dressings		44
Mobility		45
Hygiene		46
Preparation – hot drink, simple snack		47
Feeding		48
Environment		49
Washing and grooming		50
Bathing or shower		51
Chair		52
Wheelchair		53
Bladder function		54
Bowel function		55
Medication		56
Treatment		57
Management of household		58
Emotional health		59
Sleep		60
Time up during day		61

Life Satisfaction Profile

How often do you do the following activities?

1 Reading books, newspapers or magazines	62
2 Taking walks	63
3 Sewing, knitting or crocheting	64
4 Watching TV or listening to the radio	65
5 Visiting friends or relations at their home	66
6 Making dinner for friends or relatives	67
7 Attending cinema, theatre or sporting events	68
8 Social games (chess, dominoes, cards, disco)	69
9 Fishing, hunting, golf, bowling or other sport	70
10 Playing a musical instrument	71
11 Hobbies (stamp collecting, model-making, etc.)	72

	code		code		code
Every day	6	Once a week	4	Once a month	2
2 or 3 times per week	5	About twice a month	3	A couple of times a year	1
				Never	0
				No information	X

12 Do you belong to any club or organisations which hold regular meetings?	Yes	
	No	73
	No information	

13 What are these organisations, and how often do they meet? (see list)

14 How often did you attend meetings? (see list)

---

15 Were you an officer or have any special responsibilities such as chairman
or member of a committee? (see list)

---

16 About how much time all together (a week or a month) did you devote to
your organisation, including all meetings, functions and other work done?

List

Organisation	Frequency of meetings	Time spent	How often patient attended	Positions held and duties	
					74
					75
					76
					77

1	2	3
Agree	Disagree	Undecided

Check boxes from right to left with a diagonal line with an X
score one point.

17 As I grow older, things seem better than I thought they would be	1	2	3	78
18 I have had more chances in life than most of the people I know	1	2	3	79
19 This is the dreariest time of my life	1	2	3	80
20 I am just as happy now as when I was younger	1	2	3	81
21 My life could be happier than it is now	1	2	3	82
22 These are the best years of my life	1	2	3	83
23 Most of the things I do are boring or monotonous	1	2	3	84

24 I expect some interesting and pleasant things to happen to me in the future

25 The things I do today are as interesting to me as they ever were

26 I feel old and somewhat tired

27 As I look back on my life I am fairly well satisfied

28 I would not change my past even if I could

29 I like to take an interest in my appearance

30 I have made plans for things I'll be doing in a month or a year from now

31 When I think back over my life, I didn't get most of the important things I wanted

32 Compared to other people, I get down in the dumps too often

33 I've got pretty much what I expected out of life

34 In spite of what people say, the life of the average person is getting worse not better

				85
				86
				87
				88
				89
				90
				91
				92
				93
				94
				95

96 97

Total Score   LS1 Boxes with an X score one point

Patient Service Checklist (discharge)

Name:_____ I am pleased that you are now able to leave hospital, before you go could I please ask some questions about your stay in hospital?

	True	Not True	Not applic-able	
35 The radio or television was noisy	0	1	X	98
36 My bed bath was not given to me when I wanted it	0	1	X	99
37 The nurse was usually in a hurry	0	1	X	100
38 Couldn't get anything from nurse for pain	0	1	X	101
39 The nurse was prompt in answering my call	1	0	X	102
40 Food trays were removed as soon as I was finished	1	0	X	103
41 Thermometer left in too long	0	1	X	104
42 Didn't see nurse often enough	0	1	X	105
43 My bedpan or commode was removed promptly	1	0	X	106
44 My food was served at the right temperature	1	0	X	107
45 Nurse or assistants left me with clean towels	1	0	X	108
46 My meals were served as I had ordered	1	0	X	109
47 Drinking water was changed regularly	1	0	X	110
48 Other patients made disturbing noises	0	1	X	111
49 Nurse left before I could ask her questions	0	1	X	112
50 Had to wait too long for a bedpan	0	1	X	113
51 The nurses offered to stay with me when I was first allowed up	1	0	X	114
52 The nurses fed me when I needed help	1	0	X	115
53 My room was comfortable to sleep in	1	0	X	116
54 I was not propped up, making it hard to enjoy my meal	0	1	X	117
55 The nurses never told me how they were going to care for me	0	1	X	118
56 The nurses let me do things at my own speed	1	0	X	119
57 The nurses offered to bathe me when I needed help	1	0	X	120

	True	Not True	Not applicable	
58 Light was too bright when I tried to sleep	0	1	X	121
59 The hallways near my room were fairly quiet	1	0	X	122
60 Nurses seemed very interested in me	1	0	X	123
61 Bathroom was not clean	0	1	X	124
62 My bath, meal or rest period was interrupted by treatment	0	1	X	125
63 If I felt bad, I was not asked to do anything I didn't want to do	1	0	X	126
64 I was woken to have my temperature taken	0	1	X	127
65 Was not served drinks after I requested them	0	1	X	128
66 In general, my room was neat and tidy	1	0	X	129
67 The nurses wouldn't tell me what was wrong with me	0	1	X	130
68 My food was cold when served	0	1	X	131
69 The nurses were very nice to me	1	0	X	132
70 The nurses were with me fairly often	1	0	X	133
71 Bed was not changed often enough	0	1	X	134
72 Patients near me were fairly quiet	1	0	X	135
73 Nurse did not wash and rub my back well	0	1	X	136
74 The nurse was not prompt in answering my call	0	1	X	137
75 Air in my room was always fresh	1	0	X	138
76 I didn't get medicine when I requested it	0	1	X	139
77 The nurses take their time with me	1	0	X	140
78 My bandage or dressing was too tight	0	1	X	141
79 Bedpan was brought to me promptly	1	0	X	142
80 I was given a wheelchair when I asked for one	1	0	X	143

Additional comments:

81 No. of days in acute hospital   144 ☐☐ 145

82 No. of days in a community hospital   146 ☐☐ 147

83 No. of days in a nursing unit   148 ☐☐ 149

84 Discharged to: Home   = 1
                  Part III   = 2   ☐ 150
                  NHS hospital   = 3
                  Private home   = 4
                  Others   = 5

Appendix IV

Criteria list for use with Nursing Dependency Index

Code	Function	Level of performance
1	Bed	● Able to rise and return to bed without help of any kind, either from other person, or prescribed aids.
2		● Able to rise and return to bed using prescribed aids, but without human assistance. (Does not exclude acceptance of occasional help for reasons other than necessity.)
3		● Requires the assistance of one person, to rise and return to bed. May also use aids.
4		● Dependent on the assistance of two persons, to rise and return to bed.
5		● Bedfast. Unable to rise, even with assistance of two persons, for any purpose.
1	Dressing	● Able to dress without help of any kind, either from other person or prescribed aids.
2		● Able to dress using prescribed aids, but without human assistance.
3		● Requires the assistance of one person to dress. May also use aids.
4		● Requires the help of two persons to dress. ● Cannot help in any stage of the procedure.
5		● Bedfast. Bedwear only. Changed by others as necessary.
1	Walking (starting from a chair)	● Able to walk throughout house, from one room to another, without help of any kind, either from other person or prescribed aids. Also, able to negotiate steps or stairs.
2		● Able to walk throughout house, from one room to another, as required, using prescribed aids, but without human

Code	Function	Level of performance
		assistance. Manages to negotiate a few steps or short flight of stairs with difficulty.
3		● Requires the assistance of one person to walk from one room to another. Can negotiate a few steps, but not stairs.
4		● Requires the help of two persons to walk a few paces. Cannot manage steps or stairs.
5		● Bedfast.
1	Toileting	● Able to use toilet without help of any kind, either from other person or prescribed aids.
2		● Able to use toilet with dependence on prescribed aids, but without human assistance.
3		● Requires the assistance of one person, either to go to toilet, and/or to complete function, cleansing operation, adjust clothing, handwashing.
4		● Requires the assistance of two persons to go to toilet, and to complete function.
5		● Bedfast. Bedpan or commode brought to bedside.
1	Provision of meal	● Able to prepare adequate meals, hot drinks, and handle utensils, crockery, cutlery, without help of any kind.
2		● Able to prepare adequate meals, hot drinks, and manipulate utensils, crockery, cutlery, using kitchen aids.
3		● Dependent on one other person or service for provision of main meals. Food brought prepared. Able to reheat as necessary.
4		● Dependent on household arrangements for provision of meals. Not able to provide meal for self.
5		● Bedfast. Meals provided.
1	Feeding	● Able to set table or tray with crockery, cutlery, and take meal without help of any kind, either from other person or aids.
2		● Able to set table or tray with crockery, cutlery and take meal, using prescribed aids.

Code	Function	Level of performance
3		● Requires the assistance of one person to set table or tray, food may require to be cut into manageable portions. Can then use cutlery.
4		● Dependent on household arrangements for table or tray setting. May require to have food cut, and some help given with feeding.
5		● Bedfast. Dependent on arrangements pertaining to situation.
1	Control of environment for comfort and safety	● Able to manipulate door knobs, open and shut doors, adjust gas and electric switches, water taps, television controls, independent of other person, or aids.
2		● Makes use of special aids and devices to retain independence in the above areas.
3		● Dependent on one other person for adjusting of heating, lighting, turning taps, television controls. Physically unable to perform manoeuvres.
4		● Environmental control not individual responsibility. May accept these services as part of household routine.
5		● Bedfast. Dependent on others for comfort and safety.
1	Washing, grooming, and bathing	● Able to wash hands and face without assistance, also clean teeth, brush and comb hair, shave (male), attend to nails. Able to bath or shower safely without supervison.
2		● Able to wash hands and face, using prescribed aids, but without human assistance. Grooming also at same level. Bathing or showering accomplished safely using prescribed aids.
3		● Requires the assistance of one person to wash hands and face. This may be to take him/her to wash-basin, or bringing equipment. Able to perform daily ablutions. Help with grooming. Bathing or showering requires the help of one person.
4		● Washing and grooming requires two persons to assist. Bathing also requires the assistance of two persons.

Code	Function	Level of performance
5		● Bedfast. Washing and bathing requires to be carried out in bed, by one or more persons.
1	Chair	● Able to sit down in chair and rise up throughout day as necessary, without help of any kind, either from other person or aids.
2		● Able to sit down in chair and rise up throughout day as necessary, using prescribed aids, but without human assistance.
3		● Requires the assistance of one person to sit down and rise up as necessary. May also use aids.
4		● Dependent on the assistance of two persons to sit down and rise up from chair.
5		● Bedfast.
1	Wheelchair	● No wheelchair required.
2		● Able to manoeuvre wheelchair, apply and release brake, without help of any kind, either from other person or aids, indoors.
3		● Requires the assistance of one person to manoeuvre wheelchair and wheeling, indoors or out.
4		● Requires the assistance of two persons to manoeuvre wheelchair, for wheeling, managing ramp, steps, indoors or out.
5		● Bedfast.
1	Bladder function	● Has full control of bladder function.
2		● Good control of bladder function, but may have occasional lapse.
3		● Weak control of bladder function. Day and/or night lapse. Able to use toilet between lapses.
4		● Incontinent − up − may use protective measures. Frequent changing necessary.
5		● Bedfast. Incontinent. Requires frequent changing.
1	Bowel function	● Has full control of bowel function.

Code	Function	Level of performance
2		● Good control of bowel function, but may have occasional lapses.
3		● Weak control of bowel function. Day or night lapses.
4		● Incontinent. Up during day. Protective measures used. Changing is necessary.
5		● Bedfast. Incontinent. Changing required.
1	Medication	● No medication required. (Does not exclude use of laxative.)
2		● Capable of taking prescribed medication without supervision by other person.
3		● Taking prescribed medication requires supervision by relative.
4		● Medication supervised by district nurse.
5		● Bedfast. Medicine given at bedside. (Medicine round if residential care.)
1	Treatment	● No treatment required.
2	includes skin care dressings injections enemata	● Treatment such as may be carried out independently, with minimum supervision, or able to carry out own treatment under regular supervision of district nurse.
3	suppositories passive exercise	● Treatment carried out in out-patient department, or doctor's sugery.
4	physiotherapy ot, chiropody	● Treatment carried out by district nurse. Home visit.
5		● Bedfast. Nursing staff, if residential home.
1	Advice and guidance	● Does not feel the need for advice or guidance. No problems.
2	(sought or given)	● Able to make contact with advice giving agencies, if necessity arises.
3		● Relies on family members, friends or neighbours to make contact with advice-giving agencies, e.g. GP, HV, social worker, if necessity arises.
4		● In regular contact with advice-giving agencies.
5		● Not capable of seeking advice or guidance on own behalf. Totally dependent.

Code	Function	Level of performance
1	Communication speech and comprehension	● Powers of speech and comprehension unaffected. No difficulty in communication.
2		● Power of speech impaired, but capable of making him/herself understood. Comprehends what is said. Communication only slight problem.
3		● Power of speech impaired to extent that he/she is incomprehensible to those unfamiliar with defect. Comprehends what is said. Communication difficult.
4		● Power of speech absent. Communication possible on simple level through signs and writing. Understands simple commands.
5		● Unable to communicate through speech or any other channel.
1	Management of household tasks, shopping, laundry	● Able to carry out light household tasks without assistance of any kind, although may make arrangements for laundry and shopping.
2		● Able to carry out light household tasks, using adaptations or aids. Arrangements for laundry and shopping.
3		● Is dependent on one other person in household for management of daily tasks. Not specific role.
4		● Is dependent on community help for management of household tasks, shopping, laundry.
5		● Bedfast. Dependent on others, according to situation.
1	Emotional health in relation to condition	● Residual disability, if any, slight. Is not restricted in any activities. Well adjusted.
2		● Able to cope with residual disability and over-come difficulties. Good adjustment made.
3		● Requires and responds to encouragement, to cope with residual disability. Nervous disposition.
4		● Anxious, easily discouraged, requires constant reassurance and attention.
5		● Mood tends to depression, tearful, labile.

Code	Function	Level of performance
1	Sleep	● Sleeps well without sedation (own report).
2		● Sleeps well with sedation (own report).
3		● Wakes once or twice during night for toilet purposes. Able to attend to own requirements.
4		● Requires attention during night for toilet purposes. Able to sleep well afterwards.
5		● Poor sleep pattern, difficulty in falling asleep or wakes early.
1	Time up during	● Able to be up all day. 10 hours.
2	day	● Able to be up most of day. Retires to bed early. 6 – 10 hours.
3		● Able to be up morning to early afternoon. 3 – 6 hours.
4		● Up for short time. 0 – 3 hours.
5		● Bedfast.

Appendix V

Nursing audit chart review schedule

Name of patient: _____

       (Last)   (First)

I Application and execution of doctor's legal orders

	Yes	No	Uncertain	Total
1 Medical diagnosis complete	7	0	3	
2 Orders complete	7	0	3	
3 Orders current	7	0	3	
4 Orders promptly executed	7	0	3	
5 Evidence that nurse understood cause and effect	7	0	3	
6 Evidence that nurse took health history into account	7	0	3	
TOTALS (42)		0		☐

II Observation of symptoms and reactions

	Yes	No	Uncertain	Total
7 Related to course of above disease(s) in general	7	0	3	
8 Related to course of above disease(s) in patient	7	0	3	
9 Related to complications due to therapy (each medication and each procedure)	7	0	3	
10 Vital signs	7	0	3	
11 Patient to his condition	7	0	3	
12 Patient to his course of disease(s)	5	0	2	
TOTALS (40)		0		☐

III Supervision of the patients

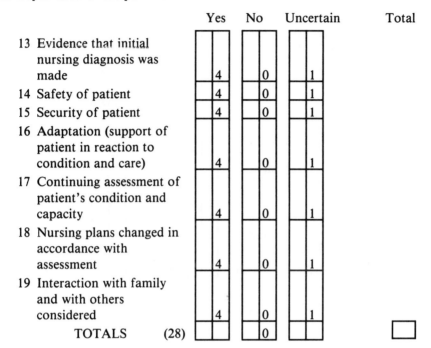

	Yes	No	Uncertain	Total
13 Evidence that initial nursing diagnosis was made	4	0	1	
14 Safety of patient	4	0	1	
15 Security of patient	4	0	1	
16 Adaptation (support of patient in reaction to condition and care)	4	0	1	
17 Continuing assessment of patient's condition and capacity	4	0	1	
18 Nursing plans changed in accordance with assessment	4	0	1	
19 Interaction with family and with others considered	4	0	1	
TOTALS (28)		0		

IV Supervision of those participating in care (except the doctor)

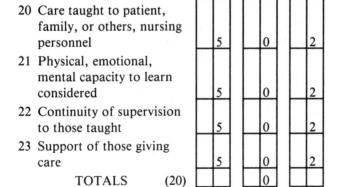

	Yes	No	Uncertain	Total
20 Care taught to patient, family, or others, nursing personnel	5	0	2	
21 Physical, emotional, mental capacity to learn considered	5	0	2	
22 Continuity of supervision to those taught	5	0	2	
23 Support of those giving care	5	0	2	
TOTALS (20)		0		

V Reporting and recording

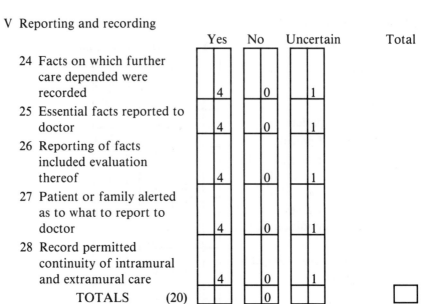

	Yes	No	Uncertain	Total
24 Facts on which further care depended were recorded	4	0	1	
25 Essential facts reported to doctor	4	0	1	
26 Reporting of facts included evaluation thereof	4	0	1	
27 Patient or family alerted as to what to report to doctor	4	0	1	
28 Record permitted continuity of intramural and extramural care	4	0	1	
TOTALS (20)		0		

VI Application and execution of nursing procedures and techniques

	Yes	No	Uncertain	Does not apply
Administration and/or supervision of medications	2	0	0.5	2
Personal care (bathing, oral hygiene, skin, nail care, shampoo)	2	0	0.5	2
Nutrition (including special diets)	2	0	0.5	2
Fluid balance plus electrolytes	2	0	0.5	2
Elimination	2	0	0.5	2
Rest and sleep	2	0	0.5	2
Physical activity	2	0	0.5	2
Irrigations (including enemas)	2	0	0.5	2
Dressings and bandages	2	0	0.5	2
Formal exercise programme	2	0	0.5	2

	Yes	No	Uncertain	Does not apply
Rehabilitation (other than formal exercise)	2	0	0.5	2
Prevention of complications and infections	2	0	0.5	2
Recreation, diversion	2	0	0.5	2
Clinical procedures — urinalysis, B/P	2	0	0.5	2
Special treatments (e.g. care of tracheotomy, use of oxygen, colostomy or catheter care, etc.)	2	0	0.5	2
Procedures and techniques taught to patient	2	0	0.5	2
TOTALS		0		

TOTAL

VII Promotion of physical and emotional health by direction and teaching

	Yes	No	Uncertain	Does not apply
Plans for medical emergency evident	3	0	1	3
Emotional support to patient	3	0	1	3
Emotional support to family	3	0	1	3
Teaching promotion and maintenance of health	3	0	1	3
Valuation of need for additional resources (eg spiritual, social service, home help service, physio or occupational therapy)	3	0	1	3
Action taken in regard to needs identified	3	0	1	3
TOTALS		0		

TOTAL

TOTAL SCORE

FINAL SCORE

Part III Audit Results

All entries to be completed by a nursing audit committee member

Record reflects service as:

Excellent (161 – 200)   Good   (121 – 160)   Incomplete (81 – 120)

☐   (   )   ☐   (   )   ☐   (   )

Poor   (41 – 80)   Unsafe   (0 – 40)

☐   (   )   ☐   (   )

Record did not permit appraisal ☐ Why?

Remarks (including criticisms/questions pertinent to policy procedures, practices as shown in Parts I and II):

_____   _____

Signature of Nursing Audit Committee   Date:
member who reviewed the record

Appendix VI

Letter to accompany staff questionnaire – phase 1

Staff Letter – Phase 1

Dear
Enclosed is a rather detailed questionnaire which looks at how nurses feel about their work, how they work, and about the place in which they work. I would be very grateful if you would complete the questionnaire, without discussing it with your colleagues, and hand it back to ... [senior nursing officer].

The purpose of the questionnaire is to both find out about any changes which could be made at ... [study hospital] and to use it as a measure in a couple of years to see if any of your views change after I start as nursing officer in September.

You do not need to write your name on the questionnaire, and your replies will be confidential.

I am really looking forward to taking up the post, and to getting to know you all. The results of the questionnaire will be shared with all of the staff when we begin to look at the hospital's work, and decide together on how we can make ... [study hospital] even better than it already is.

With many thanks,

Appendix VII

Letter to accompany consumer questionnaire

Dear

As part of our continued attempts to look at the service provided at ... [study hospital], and to improve them, we are seeking the opinions of the local people.

Enclosed is a short questionnaire, and it would be greatly appreciated if you would complete it and return it to me in the stamped addressed envelope provided.

Your replies will be treated confidentially, and will be used to consider how we should proceed in improving the service we provide.

Thank you very much, in advance, for your help and support.

Appendix VIII

Nursing officer job description

Job Description

Title: Nursing Officer

Department: Nursing

Accountable to: Director of Nursing Services

Overall objectives:
1. To be administratively accountable for ... Hospital and Community Nursing Services
2. To be available to the DNS and Nursing staff to provide expertise and advice on all clinical nursing matters
3. To be a resource for the introduction, teaching and demonstration of appropriate methods of nursing care.
4. To develop philosophies of care and to build a framework which can be used as a model for future nursing care
5. To be available as a resource on clinical nursing matters for nurses in the District

Key result areas:
1. To assess and inform the DNS of changes in clinical nursing practice with implications for the Community Unit
2. To ensure the involvement and development of appropriate unit nurses in research schemes and act as a resource for information
3. To establish a climate in which individual skills, knowledge and attitudes of nursing staff are developed to prepare them to make an effective contribution and professional input within their working teams
4. To participate in community senior management meetings
5. To be a member of the Nursing Process Group

	6.	To participate as required in nursing standards groups/education committees as appropriate
Working relationships:	1.	Monitored by the District Clinical Practice Nurse
	2.	Service giving relationship to nursing services.
Profile:	1.	To provide an efficient in-patient/out-patient nursing service at ... Hospital.
	2.	To co-ordinate the primary care team attached to the general practitioners at ...
	3.	To be available to the Director of Nursing Services and nursing staff to provide expertise and advice on all clinical nursing matters.

Appendix IX

Job descriptions developed in phase 2 for qualified nurses

Job title:	Primary nurse
Grade:	Staff nurse
Responsible to:	Senior nurse
Monitored by:	Senior nurse
Hours:	37.5 per week

Overall objectives:

1. To assess, plan, implement and evaluate care for patients allocated to him/her.
2. To be responsible for the implementation of care by associate nurses.
3. To act as associate nurse to other primary nurses in their absence.

Key result areas:

1. To give a high standard of direct care to patients.
2. To supervise care assistants.
3. To document accurately the four stages of the nursing process.
4. To communicate effectively with all of the members of the multidisciplinary clinical team.
5. To be responsible for total care and therefore be available out-of-hours in the event of the need for major changes in the care plan.
6. To be aware of current advances in clinical care.
7. To participate actively in nursing research.
8. To develop close relationships with the patient and his/her family.
9. To contribute towards an efficient and harmonious environment in the unit.
10. To maintain patients case notes.
11. To ensure that the unit is clean and tidy.
12. To take all measures to ensure the safety of patients, visitors and staff and report all incidents/accidents/hazards to the senior

nurse and community personnel department
using the correct procedure.

13. To ensure that all equipment is maintained
and used safely.

14. To ensure care and custody of patients'
property and valuables in line with the
agreed policies.

15. To attend courses/in-service training as
required.

16. Any other duties as directed by the senior
nurse.

Job title:	Associate nurse
Grade:	Staff nurse
Responsible to:	Senior nurse
Monitored by:	Senior nurse
Overall objectives:	To implement and evaluate nursing care planned by primary nurses.
Key result areas:	

1. To give a high standard of direct care to
patients.

2. To supervise care assistants.

3. To liaise with off-duty primary nurses as
appropriate.

4. To document care accurately.

5. To communicate effectively with all of the
members of the multidisciplinary team.

6. To be aware of current advances in clinical
care.

7. To participate actively in nursing
research.

8. To contribute towards an efficient and
harmonious environment in the unit.

9. To ensure that the unit is clean and tidy.

10. To take all measures to ensure the safety of
patients, visitors and staff and report all
incidents/accidents/hazards to the senior
nurse and community personnel department
using the correct procedure.

11. To ensure that all equipment is maintained
and is used safely.

12. To ensure care and custody of patients' property and valuables in line with the agreed policies.
13. To attend courses/in-service training as required.
14. Any other duties as directed by the senior nurse.

Appendix X

Patient referral form

Referral form	*Name of patient* *Age*
	Hospital/Unit patient at present time
	Person making request
	Date: *Time:*

To be filled in by nurse

1. Complete diagnoses and any other conditions _____

2. If surgery performed:-
   Surgical procedures and dates _____

3. State of wound (healed, draining, infected, sutures) _____

4. Has patient been informed of diagnosis? ☐ Yes ☐ No
   If NO, what has he/she been told _____

5. Prognosis: _____

6. How much longer would you consider it necessary for this patient to be hospitalised? _____

7. State reason for requesting transfer to [study hospital]

8. Does the patient's GP plan to visit daily? ☐ Yes ☐ No
   If not: a) How often _____
             b) Will they contact a ... GP _____

9. At time of discharge from ... Hospital is it expected that the patient will be able to:
   Return to own or relative's home ☐ Yes ☐ No
   Need permanent institutional placement ☐ Yes ☐ No

10. What are the patient's reaction to referral?

‾‾‾‾‾	‾‾‾‾‾	‾‾‾‾‾	‾‾‾‾‾
Indifferent	Objects	Accepts	Eager

11. Has this patient been evaluated for home care?   ☐ Yes ☐ No
    If NO, why not? _____

12. Is patient known to Social Services? ☐ Yes ☐ No
    Signed _____

Nursing needs

1. Indicate extent and type of care given _____

2. Degree of responsibility patient assumes for own care _____

3. Concerns patient expresses *re* self, family, finances, other _____

4. Is there any information you can share with us about family or visitors that would be helpful in his care at Burford? _____

Social needs

1. Does patient have a home to go to? _____

2. Does patient have type of home, help, family, etc. that would allow his returning to home? _____

3. Does family want patient if patient lives with others? _____
Please add any additional relevant data which would affect discharge plans: _____
On transfer from hospital to ... please forward patient's diet sheet.

For [study hospital]'s use:
Accepted:
Not accepted:
Reasons:

Appendix XI

Home assessment

Name	Address
D.o.B. Age	
Next of kin	Tel.
Address	GP
	Consultant
	District nurse/health visitor
Tel.	
Source of ref.	Reason for ref.
Medical problems:	
Current medication	
Type of accommodation and facilities:	
Support Systems	
Relatives/friends, etc.	Other agencies
Obstacles to self-care/independence at home	
Other relevant information	
Recommendations:	
Signature of assessing nurse Date	

Appendix XII

Patient Assessment Form: Basic Data

___

Community	
Hospital	
Day unit	

Hospital/Unit

Date of admission   Date of assessment   Nurse

Male ☐ Age ☐   Surname   Forenames
Female ☐
Date of birth   Prefers to be addressed
as:

Single/Married/Widowed/Other

Address of usual residence

Type of accommodation

Family/others at this residence

Next of kin   Name   Address

                 Relationship   Tel. No.

Significant others
(incl. relatives/dependants/
visitors/helpers/neighbours

Support services

Occupation

Religious beliefs and relevant
practices

Significant life crises

Patient's perception of current
health status

_____

Family's perception of patient's
health status

_____

Reason for admission

_____

Medical information (e.g. diagnosis, past history, allergies)	Weight _____ Urine _____ SG. _____ ALB _____ Temp _____ Pulse _____ B.P. Resp
Discharge arrangements: (to be completed on admission) Main source for assessment:	Projected date of discharge

Significant others interviewed: Yes/No   Arrangements discussed with:

If YES, Details of interview	Relatives _____ Others _____ Home help _____ D/N _____ H/V _____ Social worker

AL	Usual routines: What he/she can and cannot Do independently	Patient's problems (Actual/potential) (P) = Potential
Maintaining a Safe environment		
Communicating		
Breathing		
Eating and drinking		
Eliminating		
Personal cleansing and dressing		
Controlling body temperature		
Mobilising		

Assessment of Activities of Living   Date

Working and playing
Expressing sexuality
Sleeping
Dying

Appendix XIII

Information letter to participants in interdisciplinary workshops – phase 3

Dear

The arrangements for the series of workshops are almost finalised, and I write to give you more information.

Firstly, the nature of the workshops is very open, and the overall purpose is to explore the effects of how we work as both individuals, and as a team, on the consumer of Primary care. The emphasis therefore is on the CLIENT'S perceptions, and how we can learn from this, rather than on how we view each other (although the latter will inevitably need to be considered). This approach is innovative, and this series of workshops are very much pilots for future work.

Your first three sessions will commence at 1.30 pm, while the last session will be in the evening.

The organisation of the sessions involves a colossal amount of work, and the costs incurred are considerable. Given this, and the fact that we hope to generate both ideas about future sessions and generalisation about team work, it is most important that all participants attend all of their scheduled sessions.

... and the guest facilitators feel that the outcome of the sessions will be very valuable to you as an individual and to all of us as a team. We look forward to seeing you in May.

Yours sincerely,

Alan Pearson
Nursing Officer

A SERIES OF PATIENT-CENTRED COMMUNICATION
WORKSHOPS
for General practitioners, District Nurses, Health Visitors
and Hospital Nurses

I am currently finalising arrangements for these workshops, and write to give
you some preliminary information:

1. The purpose of the workshops is to explore communication between
    patient and practitioners and consider the effects of the workings of the
    'teams' on the care received by patients.

2. The format of the sessions will be the same as previous sessions, i.e. role
    play between professionals and actor patients followed by discussion.

3. Organisation of the sessions will be as follows:

    A total number of sixteen health workers will participate: four general
    practitioners, four district nurses, four health visitors and four hospital
    nurses.

    (a) The first four sessions will be single disciplines.
    (b) Sessions 5 – 8 will be mixed disciplines – i.e. one of each of the four
        disciplines.
    (c) Sessions 9 – 10 will consist of eight people – two for each discipline.
    (d) The final sessions will take the form of an evaluative discussion, for
        all sixteen participants.

    Thus each participant must be prepared to attend four sessions – one
    for his/her own discipline, one small mixed group, one large mixed
    group and the final session.

4. Group leadership: . . . will act as co-facilitator for each session, and one
    of the following will act as the other, depending on the group:

    (a) . . .
    (b) . . .
    (c) . . .
    (d) . . .

5. Cost: The series is being sponsored by . . . and several industrial firms
    and thus there are no costs for the course itself. Drinks, etc., will,
    however, have to be paid for by the participants.

    I enclose a preliminary list of the dates *your* sessions will be held. Could
you contact me *urgently* if any of these dates are inconvenient, so that I can
reorganise if possible.

Appendix XIV

Questionnaire administered to participants on interdisciplinary workshop – phase 3

Patient-centred communication workshops:
Participants' Questionnaire

It would be very helpful for the running of future workshops to know your response to what took place. Could you therefore answer all of the questions below as fully as you feel able. You do not need to sign this questionnaire.

1. How did you feel about the workshops BEFORE you came?
2. How did you feel about the workshops AFTER you had participated in them?
3. What did you think you learnt from:
    (a) the single disciplinary session?
    (b) the multidisciplinary sessions?
4. Can you point to any ideas that were confirmed or contradicted by your experience in the workshops, about:
    (a) your role?
    (b) others' roles?
    (c) patients' expectations?
    (d) other areas?
5. These were the first workshops of this kind. Do you have any recommendations which may help us in conducting any future workshops of a similar nature?

Thank you for completing this questionnaire.

Appendix XV

Letter to accompany staff questionnaire – phase 4

Staff letter – Phase 4

Dear

As we discussed at the last get-together, here is the questionnaire we all agreed to complete so that we can see if there has been any changes in our views over the last couple of years. It is really important that the questions are answered immediately, and not thought about for days before letting pen touch paper! As the questionnaire is supposed to find out how each of us feels as an individual, it is inappropriate to discuss how to answer each question with each other.

The answers are anonymous, and therefore what each of us feels will be confidential, except if we want to discuss any feelings openly in the staff group.

Have fun – and return the completed forms to me as soon as possible.

Bibliography

Abdellah F, Beland I L, Martin A and Mathergy R V (1960) *Patient Centred Approaches to Nursing*, Macmillan, New York.

Abdellah F G and Levine E (1965) *Better Patient Care Through Nursing Research*, Macmillan, New York.

Alfano G J (1969) A professional approach to nursing practice. *Nursing Clinics of North America* 4(3): 487−93.

Alfano G J (1971) Healing or caretaking − which will it be? *Nursing Clinics of North America* 6: 273−80.

Anderson E R (1973) *The Role of the Nurse*, Royal College of Nursing, London.

Archer S E, Kelly C D and Bisch S A (1984) *Implementing Change in Communities. A collaborative process*, C V Mosby, St Louis.

Argyle M (1972) *The Psychology of Interpersonal Behaviour* (2nd edition), Penguin Books, Harmondsworth.

Bailey J (1975) *Social Theory for Planning*, Routledge & Kegan Paul, London.

Bailey J T and Clause K E (1975) *Decision Making in Nursing,* C V Mosby, St Louis.

Baker D (1978) *Attitudes of Nurses to the Care of the Elderly,* unpublished PhD thesis, University of Manchester.

Barrett J (1968) *The Head Nurse − Her changing role* (2nd edition), Appleton-Century-Crofts, New York.'

Barrows H S (1971) *Simulated Patients. The development and use of a new technique in medical education,* Thomas, Illinois.

Batchelor I (1980) *The Multi-disciplinary Clinical Team − a working paper*, King's Fund, London.

Beckhard R (1969) Helping a group with planned change: a case study. *Journal of Social Issues* 15: 13−19.

Beland I L (1970) *Clinical Nursing: Pathophysiological and psychosocial approaches*, Collier-Macmillan, London.

Bell C and Roberts H (eds) (1984) *Social Researching: Politics, problems, practice*, Routledge & Kegan Paul, London.

Benne K (1966) Deliberate changing as a facilitation of growth. In Bennis W, Benne K and Chin R (1966) *The Planning of Change*, Holt, Reinhart & Winston, New York.

Bennett A E (1974) Outcome of patient care. In: Bennett A E (ed.) (1974) *Community Hospitals: Progress in development and evaluation*, Oxford Regional Hospital Board: 59−65.

Bennet J G (1980) Foreword to symposium on the self-care concept of nursing. *Nursing Clinics of North America* 15(1), W B Saunders, Philadelphia.

Bennis W, Benne K and Chin R (1966) *The Planning of Change*, Holt, Rhinehart & Winston, New York.

Berger P L (1966) *Invitation to Sociology*, Pelican Books, Harmondsworth.

Beyers M and Phillips C (1971) *Nursing Management for Patient Care*, Little, Brown, Boston.

Bhola H S (1975) The design of (educational) policy: Directing and harnessing social power for social outcomes. *Viewpoints* 51(3):2.

Binnie A (1984) The third step of the nursing process – implementation. In *A Systematic Approach to Nursing Care*, Open University Press, Milton Keynes.

Bloch D (1975) Criteria, standards, norms. *Journal of Nursing Administration*, September.

Bond S (1978) *Dilemmas in Clinical Research*. Paper presented at Northern Regional Health Authority seminar on 'Developments in Nursing', September 1976.

Bond S (1984) The second step of the nursing process – Planning. In *A Systematic Approach to Nursing Care*, Open University Press, Milton Keynes.

Bower F L (1972) *The Process of Planning Nursing Care*, C V Mosby, St Louis.

Byrne M L and Thompson L F (1978) *Key Concepts for the Study and Practice of Nursing* (2nd edition), C V Mosby, St Louis.

Campbell L (1978) *Nursing Diagnosis and Intervention in Nursing Practice*, John Wiley, New York.

Capra F (1983) *The Turning Point. Science, society and the rising culture*, Fontana, London.

Carkhuff R R (1969) The prediction of the effects of teacher–counsellor training: development of communication and discrimination selection indexes. *Counsellor Education and Supervision*.

Carr-Saunders A M and Wilson P A (1933) *The Professions*, Frank Cass, London (reprinted 1964).

Cartwright A (1964) *Human Relations and Hospital Care*, Routledge & Kegan Paul, London.

Cartwright A (1974) Studies of patients. *British Medical Bulletin*, 30 (3): 218–22.

Chapman C (1979) Sociological theory related to nursing. In Colledge M M and Jones D (eds) *Readings in Nursing*, Churchill Livingstone, Edinburgh.

Chin R (1966) The utility of systems models and developmental models for practitioners. In Bennis W, Benne K and Chin R, *The Planing of Change*, Holt, Rhinehart & Winston, New York.

Chin R and Benne K D (1976) General strategies for effecting changes. In

Bennis W, Benne K and Chin R (1966) *The Planning of Change*, Holt, Rhinehart & Winston, New York.

Christman, L (1973) The nurse clinical specialist. In Riehl J E and McVay J (eds) *Clinical Nurse specialists*. Appleton Century Crofts, New York.

Clark J (1984) Community Nursing, *Lampada* 1: 13.

Clark J M and Hockey L (1979) *Research for Nursing*, HM&M, Aylesbury.

Clarke M (1979a) Getting through the work. In Dingwall R and McIntosh J (eds) *Readings in the Sociology of Nursing*, Churchill Livingstone, Edinburgh.

Clarke M (1979b) Routinization militates against communication with patients. *Journal of Advanced Nursing* 4(1): 94−6.

Cohen G (1964) *What's Wrong with Hospitals*, Penguin Books, London.

Coser R L (1958) Authority and decision making in a hospital. *American Sociological Review* XIII: 56−64.

Coser R L (1964) *Life in the Ward*, Michigan State University Press, Michigan.

Craig J B (1976) The hospitals' internal communications project. In Revans R W, *Action Learning in Hospitals*, McGraw-Hill, London: 116−56.

Dahrendorf R (1958) Toward a theory of social conflict. *The Journal of Conflict Resolution 3* (XI.2): 170−83.

Davies C (1976) Experience of dependency and control in work: the case of nurses. *Journal of Advanced Nursing* 1(4): 273−82.

Davies C (1977) Continuities in the development of hospital nursing in Britain. *Journal of Advanced Nursing* 1(5): 479−93.

Davis F (1975) Professional socialisation as subjective experience. In Cox C and Mead A (eds), *A Sociology of Medical Practice*, Collier-Macmillan, London.

De Cecco J D (1974) *The Psychology of Learning and Instruction*, Prentice Hall, New Jersey.

Denzin N K (1970) *The Research Act in Sociology*, Butterworth, London.

Dickoff J and James P (1968) Researching research's role in theory development. *Nursing Research* 17: 204−6.

Dingwall R and McIntosh J (1979) *Readings in the Sociology of Nursing*, Churchill Livingstone, Edinburgh.

Donnison D V (1970) *Action Research*. Summary for CES governors and staff from conclusions the author drew from the SSRC conference on action research held at the University of York, 3−5 July 1970 (unpublished).

Donovan J (1971) Is the delivery system of health care the crucial problem in nursing service? *Journal of Nursing Administration*, March/April.

Doughty D B & Mash N J (1977) *Nursing Audit*, Davis, Philadelphia.

Duberley J (1977) How will the change strike me and you? *Nursing Times* 73 (45): 1736−8.

Dunn H L (1961) *High Level Wellness*, R W Beaty, Arlington, VA.

Eardley A et al. (1975) Health education by chance. *International Journal of Health Education* 18 (1): 19−25.

Elhart D, Firsich S C, Gragg S H, and Rees O M (1978) *Scientific Principles in Nursing* (8th edition), C V Mosby, St Louis.

Elpern E H (1977) Structural and organisational supports for primary nursing. *Nursing Clinics of North America* 11:2, June.

Engel G L (1962) The nature of disease and the care of the patient: the challenge of humanism and science in medicine. *Rhode Island Medical Journal* 45: 245−51.

Faulkner A (1981) Aye, there's the rub. *Nursing Times*, 19 February: 332−6.

Field D (1972) Disability as social deviance. In Friedson E and Corber J, *Medical Men and their Work*, Aldine Atherton, New York.

Flintstead W J (ed.) (1970) *Qualitative methodology. Firsthand involvement with the social world*, Markham, Chicago.

Friedrichs J (1979) *Methoden Emirischer Socialforschung*, Rourohlt, Hamburg: 370−3.

Friedson E (1970) *Professional Dominance. The social structure of health care*, Aldine, Chicago.

Friedson E (1975) *The Profession of Medicine*, Dodds, Mead & Co., New York.

Garraway W M, Akhtar A J, Prescott R J and Hockey L (1980) Management of acute stroke in the elderly: preliminary results of a controlled trial. *British Medical Journal* 280: 1040−3.

Glaser B and Strauss A (1967) *The Discovery of Grounded Theory*, Weidenfeld & Nicolson, London.

Glaser B G and Strauss A L (1970) The discovery of grounded theory. In Filstead W J (ed.), *Qualitative Methodology: First-hand involvement with the social world*, Markham, Chicago.

Goffman E (1963) *Stigma*, Penguin Books, Harmondsworth.

Goffman E (1968) *Asylums*, Penguin Books, Harmondsworth.

Gonzalez F (1981) How should nursing be managed below the level of director of nursing services? *Nursing Times*, 77: 14.

Goss M E W (1963) Patterns of bureaucracy among hospital staff physicians. In Friedson E, *The Hospital in Modern Society*, The Free Press, Toronto.

Great Britain, Ministry of Health (Salmon Committee) (1966) *Report of the Committee on the Senior Nursing Staff Structure*, HMSO, London.

Gross N, Ciaquinta J and Bernstein H (1971) *Implementing Organizational Innovations*, Basic Books, New York.

Hall D J (1978) what nurse don't see, she don't worry about − or the use of observation in hospital research, *Nursing Times*, 74 (49) (Occasional Paper 34): 137−40.

Hall L E (1964) *Project Report. The Solomon and Betty Loeb Center at Montefiore Hospital*, The Center, New York.

Hall L E (1966) Another view of nursing care and quality. In Straub M and Parker K (eds) (1966) *Continuity of Patient Care: The role of nursing* Catholic University of America Press, Washington DC.

Hall L E (1969) The Loeb Center for Nursing and Rehabilitation, Montefiore Hospital and Medical Center, Bronx, NY. *International Journal of Nursing Studies* 6: 81–95.

Hall L E, Alfano G J, Figkin M and Levine H S (1975) *Longitudinal Effects of an Experimental Nursing Process*, Loeb Center for Nursing, New York.

Hannay D R (1980) Teaching interviewing with simulated patients. *Medical Education* 14: 246–8.

Harman W (1969) The nature of our changing society. Unpublished research paper, Stamford Research Institute. In Thomas J M, and Bennis N G. *Management of Change and Conflict*, Penguin Books, London, 1972.

Hawthorn P (1974) *Nurse, I Want my Mummy*, Royal College of Nursing, London.

Hegyvary S T and Haussman R K D (1976) Monitoring nursing care quality. *Journal of Nursing Administration*, 6: 9.

Helt E H and Pelikan J A (1975) Quality: Medical care's answer to Madison Avenue. *American Journal of Public Health* 65: 284–90.

Henderson V (1966) *The Nature of Nursing*, Collier-Macmillan, London.

Her Majesty's Stationery Office (1966) *Better Services for the Mentally Handicapped*, HMSO, London.

Holmlund B A (1967) *Nursing Study: Phase one*, University of Saskatchewan, Saskatoon.

Hover J and Zimmer M J (1978) Nursing quality assurance: the Wisconsin System. *Nursing Outlook*, 26: 4.

Hunt J M and Marks-Maran D J (1979) *Nursing Care Plans. The nursing process at work*, HM & M, London.

Illich I (1975) *Medical Nemesis*, Calder & Boyers, London.

James N (1984) A postscript to nursing. In Bell C & Roberts H (eds) (1984), *Social Researching: Politics, problems, practice*, Routledge & Kegan Paul, London: 125–46.

Johnson M M and Davis M L C (1975) *Problem Solving in Nursing Practice*, Wm C Brown, Iowa.

Jourard S (1971) *The Transparent Self*, D Van Nostrand, New York.

Katzmann L (1977) *Health Care in Burford*, unpublished paper, Oxford Area Health Authority.

Kings English Dictionary (1930) British Book Co., London.

Konig R (1973) Die Beobachtung. In Konig, R (ed.) (1973), *Grundlegende Methoden und Techniken der empirischen Sozialforschung*, Ferdinand Enke, Stuttgart: 1–53.

Kratz C (1977) The nursing process. *Nursing Times* 73 (23): 854–5.

Kron T (1976) *The Management of Patient Care*, W B Saunders, Philadelphia.

Lambertson E C (1953) *Nursing Team Organization and Functioning*, Columbia University Press, New York.

La Monica E L (1979) *The Nursing Process – a humanistic approach*, Addison-Wesley, California.

La Monica E L et al. (1977) Empathy training, *Nursing Mirror*, 25 August: 22–5.

Lancet, The (1981) Assessment and teaching of empathy, 14 March: 596–7.

Larkin D D and Becker B A (1977) *Problem-oriented Nursing Assessment*, McGraw-Hill, New York.

Law G (1984) Reviewing the nursing process. In *A Systematic Approach to Nursing Care*, Open University Press, Milton Keynes.

Leino A (1951) Organizing the nursing team, *American Journal of Nursing* 51, November: 665–7.

Lelean S (1973) *Ready for Report Nurse*, Royal College of Nursing, London.

Levin L. Katz A and Host E (1979) *Self Care: Lay initiatives in health*, Prodist, New York.

Lewin K (1946) Action research and minority problems, *Journal of Social Issues* 2: 34–6.

Lewis L (1968) This I believe … About the nursing process. *Nursing Outlook* 16(5): 26–9.

Luker K A (1982) *Evaluating Health Visiting Practice*, Royal College of Nursing, London.

MacGuire J M (1980) *The Expanded Role of the Nurse*, King's Fund, London.

Maguire P et al. (1978) The value of feedback in teaching interviewing skills. *Psychological Medicine* 8: 695–704.

Manthey M (1973) Primary nursing is alive and well in the hospital. *Nursing Forum* IX(1): 65.

Manthey M et al. (1970) Primary nursing. *Nursing Forum* 9(1): 64–83.

Manthey M and Kramer M S (1970) 'A dialogue on primary nursing'. *Nursing Forum* 9: 356–79.

Marram G (1979) Perspectives in nursing management. In *Primary Nursing* Vol., 1, C V Mosby, St Louis: 84–92.

Marriner Ann (1979) *The Nursing Process* (2nd edition), C V Mosby, St Louis.

Mauksch I B and Miller M H (1981) *Implementing Change in Nursing*, C V Mosby, St Louis.

Mayers M G (1972) *A Systematic Approach to the Nursing Care Plan*, Appleton-Century-Crofts, New York.

Mayers M et al. (1977) *Quality Assurance for Patient Care – Nursing perspectives*, Appleton-Century-Crofts, New York.

McConaghey R M S (1964) *The Evolution of the Cottage Hospital*. Paper presented at the South West of England Faculty of the College of General Practitioners, Torquay, 6 June.

McFarlane J K (1976) The role of research and the development of nursing theory. *Journal of Advanced Nursing* 1: 443–51.

McFarlane J (1980a) *The Multi-disciplinary Team*, King's Fund, London.

McFarlane J (1980b) *Essays on Nursing*, King's Fund, London.

McFarlane J K and Castledine G (1982) *A Guide to the Practice of Nursing Using the Nursing Process*, C V Mosby, London.

Meadows R and Hewitt C (1972) Teaching communication skills with the help of actresses and video simulation, *British Journal of Medical Education* 6: 317–22.

Mechanic D (1975) Ideology, medical technology and health care organization in modern nations, *American Journal of Public Health* 65: 241–7.

Melia K (1981) *Student Nurses' Accounts of their Work and Training – a qualitative analysis*, unpublished PhD thesis, University of Edinburgh.

Menzies I E P (1960) Nurses under stress: a social system functioning as a defence against anxiety. *International Nursing Review* 7(6): 9–16.

Metcalfe C A (1982) Patient allocation in a maternity ward: a Report of some of the findings. In Redfern S J, Sisson A R, Walker J F and Walsh P A (eds) (1982) *Issues in Nursing Research*, Macmillan, London.

Meyer V (1981) *Unpublished M.Sc. Thesis*. The Introduction of the nursing process in a long stay geriatric ward – a study of change, University of Manchester, Department of Nursing.

Miller E J and Gwynne G V (1972) *A Life Apart*, Tavistock, London.

Mitchell J R A (1984) Is nursing any business of doctors? A simple guide to the 'nursing process'. *British Medical Journal* 288: 216–19.

Moody R and Moody J (1983) *The Book of Burford*, Barracuda Books, Buckingham.

Moroney J (1966) *Facts from Figures*, Penguin Books, Harmondsworth.

Murray M (1976) *Fundamentals of Nursing*, Prentice Hall, New Jersey.

Neugarten B L, Havighirst R J and Tobin S S (1961) The measurement of life satisfaction. *Journal of Gerontology* 16: 134–43.

Neuman B (1980) The Betty Neuman health-care systems model: a total person approach to patient problems. In Riehl J P and Roy C, *Conceptual Models for Nursing Practice*, Appleton-Century-Crofts, New York.

Nie N H (1975) *Statistical Package for the Social Sciences* (2nd edition), McGraw-Hill, New York.

Norris C M (1979) Self care. *American Journal of Nursing*, March.

Norton D et al. (1962) *An Investigation of Geriatric Nursing Problems in Hospital* (reprinted 1975), Churchill Livingstone, Edinburgh.

Oddie J A, Vine S M, Hasler J C and Bennett A E (1971) The community hospital. A pilot trial. *The Lancet.* 7 August: 308–10.

Oppenheim A N (1966) *Questionnaire Design and Attitude Measurement*, Heinemann, London.

Orem D E (1966) Discussion of paper by L E Hall: Another View of nursing care equality. In Straub M and Parker K (eds), *Continuity of Patient Care: the Role of Nursing*, Catholic University of America Press, Washington DC

Orem D E (1971) *Nursing Concepts of Practice*, McGraw-Hill, New York.

Orem D E (1980) *Nursing: Concepts of Practice* (2nd edition), McGraw-Hill, New York.

Ottaway R M (1976) A change strategy to implement new norms, new style and new environment in the work organization. *Personnel Review* 5(1), Winter.

Ottaway R M (1980) *Defining the Change Agent*. Unpublished research paper, University of Manchester Institute of Technology, Department of Management Sciences.

Oxfordshire Health Authority (1978) Unpublished discussion paper on 'Burford Hospital'.

Parlett M and Hamilton D (1972) *Evaluation as Illumination: A new approach to the study of innovatory programs*. Occasional paper, University of Edinburgh, Centre for Research in the Educational Sciences.

Parsons T (1951) *The Social System*, The Free Press of Glencoe, New York.

Pavey A E (1954) *The Story of the Growth of Nursing* (3rd edition), Faber, London.

Pearson A (1983) *The Clinical Nursing Unit*, Heinemann Medical, London.

Pearson A (1984) Quality of Patient Care Scale. In Wessex Regional Health Authority (1984) *Report on Proceedings of Senior Staff seminar on Quality Assurance*, Wessex.

Pearson A and Vaughan B A (1984a) Nursing practice and the nursing process. In *A Systematic Approach to Nursing Care*, Open University Press, Milton Keynes.

Pearson A and Vaughan B A (1984b) Introducing change into nursing practice In *A Systematic Approach to Nursing Care*, Open University Press, Milton Keynes.

Pembrey S (1980) *The Ward Sister – Key to nursing*, Royal College of Nursing, London.

Pembrey S (1984) In praise of competence. *Lampada* XX(2): 12.

Perrow C (1965) Hospitals: technology, structure and goals. In March J G (ed.) *Handbook of Organizations*, Rand-McNally, Chicago.

Perrow C (1972) *Complex Organizations: A critical essay*, Scott, Foresman, Glenville, Ill.

Phaneuf M (1976) *The Nursing Audit*, Appleton-Century-Crofts, New York.

Poirer B (1975) Loeb Center: what nursing can and should be. *The American Nurse* 7(1):5.

Punton S (1983) The struggle for independence. *Nursing Times* 2 March: 29–32.

Rapaport R N (1970) Three dilemmas in action research. *Human Relations* 23(6).

Raphael W (1969) *Patients and Their Hospitals*, King's Fund, London.

Reason P and Rowan J (1981) *Human Enquiry – a sourcebook of new paradigm research*, John Wiley, Chichester.

Reihl J P and Roy C (1980) *Conceptual Models for Nursing Practice*, Appleton-Century-Crofts, New York.

Reilly D (1975) Why a conceptual framework? *Nursing Outlook* 23:9.

Revans R W (1976) *Action Learning in Hospitals* McGraw-Hill, New York.

Reynolds M (1978) No news is bad news: patients' views about communication in hospital. *British Medical Journal* 1: 1673–6.

Robson C (1973) *Experiment, Design and Statistics in Psychology*, Penguin Books, Harmondsworth.

Rogers C R (1951) *Client-centered Therapy*, Houghton Mifflin, Boston.

Rogers M E (1980) Nursing: a science of unitary man. In Reihl J P and Roy C (1980), *Conceptual Models for Nursing Practice*, Appleton-Century-Crofts, New York.

Roper N (1976) *Clinical Experience in Nurse Education*, Churchill Livingstone, Edinburgh.

Roper N (1979) Nursing based on a model of living. In Colledge M M and Jones D (eds) (1979), *Readings in Nursing*, Churchill Livingstone, Edinburgh: 81–91.

Roper N, Logan W and Tierney A J (1980) *The Elements of Nursing*, Churchill Livingstone, Edinburgh.

Roper N, Logan W, and Tierney A J (1981) *Learning to Use the Process of Nursing*, Churchill Livingstone, Edinburgh.

Roper N, Logan W, and Tierney A J (1983) *Using a Model for Nursing*, Churchill Livingstone, Edinburgh.

Roth J A (1957) Ritual and magic in the control of contagion. *American Sociological Review* 22: 310–14.

Roth J A (1974) Professionalism: the sociologist's decoy. *Sociology of Work and Occupations* 1.

Rowden R (1984) Doctors can work with the nursing process: a reply to Professor Mitchell. *British Medical Journal* 288: 219–21.

Roy C (1980) The Roy Adaptation Model. In Reihl J P and Roy C (1980) *Conceptual Models for Nursing Practice*, Appleton-Century-Crofts, New York.

Royal College of Nursing (1979a) *Interim Report – Working Committee on Standards of Nursing Care and Related Matters (England and Wales)*.

Royal College of Nursing (1979b) Discussion paper of the working party on a clinical career structure for nurses.

Royal College of Nursing (1980) (Association of Nursing Practice) *Clinical Career Structure*, unpublished paper.

Royal College of Nursing (1981). *A Structure for Nursing*, London.

Royal College of Nursing (1981) *Towards Standards*, London.

Royal Commission on the National Health Service. Report (1979) HMSO, London.

Rue E R (1974) In Bennet A E (1974) *Community Hospitals: Progress in development and evaluation*, Oxford Regional Hospital Board, Oxford: 3–6.

Rutter D R and Maguire G P (1976) History-taking for medical students – II Evaluation of a training programme. *Lancet* II: 558.

Sanders I (1960) Approaches to social change. In Bennis W, Benne K and Chin R (1966) *The Planning of Change*. Holt, Rhinehart & Winston, New York.

Sanford N (1970) Whatever happened to action research? *Journal of Social Issues* 26(4): 3–23.

Saxton D F and Hyland P A (1975) *Planning and Implementing Nursing Intervention,* C V Mosby, St Louis.

Schaffrath W B (1978) Commission leads way to joint practice for nurses and physicians. *Hospitals* 52 (14): 78–81.

Scheff T J (1972) Decision rules and types of errors and their consequences. In Friedson E and Corber J, *Medical Men and their Work*, Aldine Atherton, New York.

Scheff T J (1974) The labelling theory of mental illness. *American Sociological Review* 39: 444–52.

Schweer J E (1972) *Creative Teaching in Clinical Nursing,* C V Mosby, St Louis.

Scott D W (1979) *CETU and Action Research.* Unpublished paper, August.

Seigal S (1956) *Nonparametric Statistics for the Behavioural Sciences,* McGraw-Hill, New York.

Shaffir W, Stebbins R and Turavetz A (eds) (1980) *Fieldwork Experience*, St Martin's Press, New York.

Sjoberg K et al. (1968) *Patient Classification Study*, University of Saskatchewan, Saskatoon.

Sjoberg K and Bicknell P (1969) *A Pilot Study to Implement and Evaluate the Unit Assignment System*, University of Saskatchewan, Saskatoon.

Sjoberg K et al. (1971) Unit assignment: a patient-centered system. *Nursing Clinics of North America.*

Smuts J C (1926) *Holism and Evolution*, Macmillan, New York.

Spelman M S, Ley P and Jones C (1966) How do we improve doctor–patient communications in our hospitals? *World Hospitals* 2: 126–34.

Stannard C (1973) Old folks and dirty work: the social conditions for patient abuse in a nursing home. *Social Problems* 20: 329–42.

Steele S J and Morton D J (1978) The ward round. *Lancet* 1, (8055): 85–6.

Stein L (1978) The doctor–nurse game. In Dingwall R and McIntosh J (eds), *Readings in the Sociology of Nursing*, Churchill Livingstone, Edinburgh: 107–17.

Stevens B J (1972) Why won't nurses write nursing care plans? *Journal of Nursing Administration* 2, November/December: 6−7, 91−2.

Stockwell F (1972) *The Unpopular Patient*, Royal College of Nursing, London.

Sundeen S J et al. (1976) *Nurse−client Interaction − implementing the nursing process*, C V Mosby, St Louis.

Susman G I and Evered R D (1978) An assessment of the scientific merits of action research. *Administrative Science Quarterly* 23: 582−603.

Swaffield L (1982) Spanner in the works. *Nursing Times*, 10 November, 1049−54.

Szasz T S (1961) *The Myth of Mental Illness*. Hoeber, New York.

Szasz T S and Hollender M H (1956) Contribution to philosophy of medicine; basic models of doctor−patient relationship. *AMA Archives of Internal Medicine* 97: 585−92.

Thompson R (1960) Organizational management of conflict. In Bennis W, Benne K, and Chin R (1966) *The Planning of Change*, Holt, Rhinehart & Winston, New York.

Tierney A (1984) The first step of the nursing process − Assessment. In *A Systematic Approach to Nursing Care*, Open University Press, Milton Keynes.

Tiffany C H (1977) *Nursing, Organizational Structure and the Real Goals of Hospitals: a Correlational Study*. Unpublished PhD Study, Indiana University.

Towell D (1975) *Understanding Psychiatric Nursing*, Royal College of Nursing, London.

Towell D (1979) A social systems approach to research and change in nursing care. *International Journal of Nursing Studies* 16.

Travelbee J (1971) *Interpersonal Aspects of Nursing*, F A Davis, Philadelphia.

Treece E W and Treece J W (1977) *Elements of Research in Nursing*, C V Mosby, St Louis.

Vine S M (1974) A geriatrician's viewpoint. In Bennet A E (ed.), *Community Hospitals: Progress in development and evaluation*, Oxford Regional Hospital Board, Oxford: 45−6.

Wainwright P and Burnip S (1983) QUALPACS at Burford. *Nursing Times* 79(5): 36−8.

Walton R (1965) Two strategies of social change and their dilemmas. In Thomas R and Bennis W (1972) *Management of Change and Conflict*, Penguin Books, Harmondsworth.

Wandelt M and Ager J (1974) *Quality Patient Care Scale*. Appleton-Century-Crofts, New York.

White R (1982) The post-war reconstruction of nursing. In Redfern S J, Sisson A R, Walker J F and Walsh P A (eds), *Issues in Nursing Research*, Macmillan, London.

Whitehouse C, Morris P and Marks B (1984) The role of actors in teaching communication. *Medical Education* 18: 262–8.

Wiedenbach E (1964) *Clinical Nursing*, Springer, New York.

Williams K (1974) Ideologies of nursing: their meanings and implications. *Nursing Times*, Occasional Papers, 8 August.

Wilson J (1972) *Philosophy and Educational Research*, Windsor National Foundation for Educational Research in England and Wales.

Wood K M (1979) *Nurse – Patient Communication in an Accident Department*, Unpublished MSc Thesis, Department of Nursing, University of Manchester.

Yura H and Walsh M B (1973) *The Nursing Process*, Appleton-Century-Crofts, New York.

Zola I R (1975) Medicine as an institution of social control. In Cox C and Mead A (eds), *A Sociology of Medical Practice*, Collier-Macmillan, London.